INFERTILITY, IVF AND MISCARRIAGE

A GUIDE FOR THE GENERAL PUBLIC

Second Edition

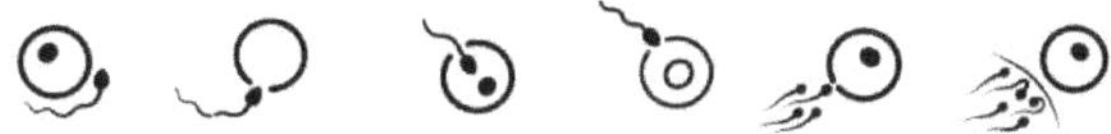

Dr Sean Watermeyer
Dr Vidya Atluri

SABGE PUBLISHING
ISBN: 978-1-8380692-6-1

We wish to thank our families, friends and indeed colleagues who have been supportive of us during the writing of this book. A special thanks to Ali for her forbearance and thanks to our consultant colleagues: Lyndon for his advice on all things embryological, Anju with regard to her review of the chapter on miscarriage, Swamy for his review of the chapter on antenatal care and finally Mr Dai Pugh for proofreading.

CONTENTS

FOREWORD

Scientific research and the gaining of new knowledge within the sphere of infertility and its treatment continues at pace. After just 5 years since the original publication, this second edition of *Infertility, IVF and Miscarriage*, brings the reader and would-be parent a straightforward guide that is up to date and current. It is amazing how much the world of fertility has changed in the last 5 years, as more evidence comes to light – a number of previous recommended interventions such as "Endometrial Scratch" or "IMSI" have gone out of favour, emphasising the importance of an up-to-date and current guide for patients wanting their own child.

We have added a number of new chapters to consolidate knowledge and incorporate the answers to questions that our patients frequently ask. This second edition benefits from the knowledge, wisdom and considerable experience of three other consultants (including a consultant embryologist) who have been kind enough to share their expertise.

There continues to be within the massive majority of us human beings a deep-seated need to replicate ourselves, to pass on a little of who we are into the next generation and beyond. It is my opinion that there is a compulsion within our nature to have children to hold, to love, and to nurture. It is as basic as the human need to love and to be loved. In a world where certainties over God, religion and afterlife are becoming ever more abstract, the certainty of living on through one's children is ever more attractive and important.

In our professional lives we have unfortunately found that there is much ignorance and misinformation banded about regarding infertility and often couples desperate to have a child are left high and dry. Advice from the internet, friends, or indeed even some medical professionals is at times confusing and on occasions erroneous. The hope is that this book, designed for the layman, provides a clearer picture and an answer to many of the questions frequently asked by couples wishing to have their own children and thus far unable to do so.

The gift of conception, and having your own child, then watching them grow up, nurturing them into the hopefully wonderful individuals they become, is indeed a rollercoaster, not to mention a huge responsibility. Boundless feelings of love, joy, tears, anger, pleasure – every conceivable (if you'll forgive the pun) emotion and completely knackering, not to mention hugely costly! It is an intrinsic part of being human and it is our wish that you, dear reader, are able to experience the joy of parenthood. This book has been written as your guide to achieve it.

Sean Watermeyer
Vidya Atluri

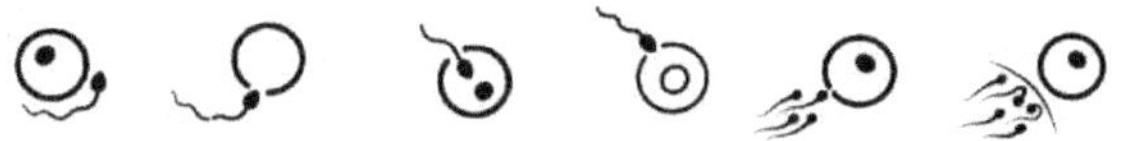

CHAPTER 1

THE PROBLEM AND WHEN TO START SEEKING ADVICE

Introduction

The aim of this short book is to empower you would-be parents with a basic understanding of the whole process of why couples cannot conceive, what must be done to investigate this, and then what is a sensible plan of action going forward, depending on the findings of investigations. More importantly we will endeavour to give you a realistic approximation of your chances of success. Please understand this is not a clinical textbook written for high flying academics. Whilst this book is certainly informative to the non-specialist doctor or nurse who regularly are confronted with patients suffering from miscarriage, PCOS, Endometriosis and infertility; it is primarily a manual written by parents who happen to also be infertility doctors; this book is written for the ordinary man and woman. It is written for heterosexuals, for homosexuals, and for loving couples of whatever persuasions who want a child of their own to love and bring up. We only hope we can do it justice and give you, the reader, the information, understanding, and courage to take things forward to achieve your dream.

How big a problem is infertility in the West?

Approximately 1 in 6 to 7 couples in the Western World

cannot have children without help. So, we guess the message is, *you are not alone*. Infertility is a common phenomenon. This, of course, accounts for why there are so many IVF units in the UK and around the world. The infertility industry is a massive one – this is why you need to make sure you have a basic understanding of the whole process. We see many couples in both the NHS and in private infertility clinics who feel that they have been misled about their inability to have children. Years go by without any active investigation or action and for sure this can make a big difference to success rates when the couple finally do get the treatment they require. Nothing gives us more satisfaction, as clinicians, to see understanding on the faces of our patients as they leave the consulting room with a basic understanding and plan of action to help them achieve their dream of becoming parents.

What is the definition of infertility?

Couples often ask the definition of infertility and the simplest answer is… if you have been trying for 1 year or more with no success you may have a problem. Some authorities state 18 months. Obviously to achieve a pregnancy it is necessary to have *regular* sex. You may laugh, but we do occasionally see couples who sit in clinic and explain that after 1 year of trying they have not managed to get pregnant, but… he lives in London and she lives in Scotland, they meet on occasional weekends and hope for the best! Therefore, the definition includes 12 to 18 months of *regular* intercourse without using any form of contraception.

How long does it take on average to get pregnant?

Do not be disheartened if the urine pregnancy test kit from the chemist is not positive after a couple of months of trying. If you take 100 women (who are 25 years old or younger) who are having regular intercourse over a 6-month time period, 60 women will have conceived (so conversely 40 women will not be pregnant). Over a 12-month time period, 85 women will have conceived. So even after a whole year of regular intercourse, 15 out of 100 perfectly healthy couples will not have managed to conceive.

So, nature often takes its time with getting people pregnant – in the majority, pregnancy is not instantaneous. The average monthly pregnancy rate of a heterosexual couple having regular intercourse is approximately 5-20% (depending on age – and more about this later). This means that for every month of trying to conceive, approximately 80-95% of the time your best efforts are not rewarded. There are occasions, of course, when pregnancy ensues after only a month or two of regular intercourse or indeed after a single act of intimacy, but as a general rule it takes the majority of couples longer. So do not be disappointed if you do not get pregnant immediately, you are in the majority.

How important is age with regard to fertility?

This is a big deal for women, not quite such a big deal for men. Men have managed to have children into their 80s and 90s, although the risk of genetic abnormality increases. For the female gender, time is of the essence. Once women get to the relatively young age of 35-37 years old, their fertility significantly reduces, such that the pregnancy rate is 85% after 2 years of trying, as opposed to 1 year of trying in women who are 25 years old.

This also occurs to a much lesser degree with men after the age of 40 years old. Probably one of the most important factors in female fertility is the age of the eggs, and this has a major influence on not only whether women get pregnant in the first place but whether they stay pregnant (in other words, the older the woman is, the older her eggs are, the greater the risk of miscarriage).

Age (years)	Approximate natural pregnancy rate per cycle of trying	Approximate miscarriage rate
20s	20-25%	10%
early 30s	15%	10-15%
35-40	10%	16-25%
early 40s	5%	30-45%
45	1%	60%

The above table indicates the approximate chances of pregnancy and miscarriage that are age related. A woman is born with a finite number of eggs (approximately 1 million per ovary), but the vast majority will degenerate over time, until there is only a fraction of the original number left (which is when she goes into menopause).

Now it's the time for hot flushes (or as the Americans say, "flashes"; somewhat unfortunate when translated into the UK equivalent). Cigarette smoking hastens this march to menopause. It is thought that it is the decline in the quality of eggs over time, as opposed to the quality of the lining (endometrium) of the womb that leads to a reduction in a woman's fertility with age. Thus, a woman can be in her 40s and still have a very good chance of having a healthy baby if she uses donor eggs from a younger woman. Men on the other hand continue to make sperm for the majority of their lives. They are not born with a set number of sperm, but produce a new batch approximately every 3 months.

How do I know how many eggs I have left in my ovaries?

There are 3 tests to determine ovarian reserve:

AMH blood test

Antral Follicle Count on ultrasound

FSH blood test

1. AMH or Anti-Mullerian Hormone. This is a simple blood test that a woman can have at any time of the month (it does not need to be taken at a particular time in a woman's cycle) that gives information on her ovarian reserve. In other words, if there are plenty of eggs in that woman's ovaries the AMH is normal or high; if the number of eggs is starting to dwindle the AMH is low. Your GP will probably not know about this and generally it is not available on the NHS, but you can have it done privately. This is a good test to have for a number of reasons:

(i)   If you are relatively young (less than 35 years old) and the AMH is normal it is reassuring that the couple have some time to play with.

(ii)   If, however, the AMH is low, then even if that woman is relatively young, the test indicates that her ovarian reserve is starting to deplete and that the sooner action is taken to help her conceive the better. Remember that approximately 1% of women will have completed their menopause by 40 years of age and we have seen and treated a number of women who were menopausal in their late 20s and early 30s – a disaster if they want their own children.

(iii)   Finally, if a couple are going for IVF then there is correlation between the AMH blood test and the number of eggs/embryos that are obtained with IVF treatment. Also, the AMH test is important in guiding the fertility doctor to determine the best dose of stimulation medication (hormonal injections which assist ovaries to grow eggs) administered in IVF cycles.

(iv) A very high AMH is a marker for a condition called Polycystic Ovarian Syndrome (PCOS) which will be discussed in a later chapter.

2. Ultrasound assessment of the ovaries. Another method of assessing ovarian reserve is to have an ultrasound scan (usually transvaginal – a small probe is placed into the vagina) that looks directly at the ovaries and counts the number of follicles (sac-like structures containing eggs). These measure anything between 2-10mm, and with progression of a woman's cycle, one of them will become dominant to release its egg. These follicles or little sacs are known as antral follicles and counting them up is known as an Antral Follicle Count or AFC for short.

The number of follicles seen on USS can be used as a marker for ovarian reserve, and hence a marker of potential menopause, as well as giving an indication as to how well a woman's ovaries will respond to medication in any given IVF cycle. Hence:

If the total AFC is:

AFC	What it means –
<4	indicates low ovarian reserve, increased risk of menopause in the next 7 years, and likely poor response to medication given to stimulate ovaries in an IVF cycle
9-19	normal
>20	indicates high ovarian reserve, and a likely excessive response to medication given to stimulate the ovaries in an IVF cycle

The AFC will inevitably get lower with increasing age until menopause is reached. If the AFC is very high, it can also be a marker for a condition called Polycystic Ovarian Syndrome (PCOS) which is covered in a later chapter.

The ultrasound scan is also very useful in ensuring you have a normal womb (uterus), normal (endometrial) lining and no abnormal cysts.

3. FSH blood test. This is a blood test that can be done by your GP in the early part of you cycle (usually day 3). Follicle Stimulating Hormone (or FSH for short) is a hormone produced by the brain that stimulates the ovary to produce an egg. If the ovaries are running out of eggs, then often the brain has to send more FSH to get the ovary to respond. So, a high FSH (>10mIU/ml) indicates low ovarian reserve, a very high FSH (>30mIU/ml) indicates menopause.

What should you do if you have a family history of early menopause (Premature Ovarian Failure)?

About 1% of women will start experiencing hot flushes, poor sleep, irregular periods and then cessation of periods before their fortieth birthday. They have likely gone into early menopause or premature ovarian failure (POF). In medical circles this is called Premature Ovarian insufficiency (POI). Then, it *may* be too late to have a baby using your own eggs, even with IVF. In most cases, the reason for POF is called "Idiopathic" – in other words nobody knows why it has happened. In other cases, there are obvious reasons, for example a past history of chemo/radiotherapy for a cancer in early childhood. If a medical cause for early menopause is not obvious, then the reason may be genetic.

It is thought that in about 10-20% of women with POF there is already a family history of it in their mother or sister.

Family history is very important:

If there is a family history of

(i)   Inherited intellectual disability or mental retardation

(ii)   Autism

(iii) Ataxia (which is abnormal balance/co-ordination/speech)

(iv) Learning disabilities, and ADHD (Attention Deficit Hyperactivity Disorder)-like symptoms, then the women may be a carrier of a genetic condition that includes Fragile X Syndrome.

Fragile X Syndrome (FXS), is the most common cause of *inherited* intellectual disability and an important genetic condition associated with early menopause is Fragile X associated Primary Ovarian Insufficiency, or FXPOI for short. Some authorities indicate that 1 in 150 women may be "carriers" of the genetic abnormality without knowing it and so be unaware of the possibility of passing it on to their children.

So, if there is a strong family history of the above, seek advice and get tested.

We guess then knowing the age at which your own mother went through the menopause is likely to give a clue for the timing of your own menopause. There is evidence that having an AMH blood test may well be a good marker of early ovarian decline even in genetic causes such as FXPOI.

If in doubt, get tested and ask for blood tests – AMH/FSH and/or an ultrasound scan.

Why is the age of the woman and her eggs important?

Up to 80-90% of eggs/embryos that are produced by a woman **over** 40 years old may be genetically abnormal – this is not to say that the woman or her partner are genetically abnormal, but that the aging process has an adverse effect on an older woman's eggs. This means natural pregnancy rates are right down and miscarriage rates are right up. This is scary stuff.

There are, of course, still women who manage to conceive and carry a baby who are 40 years old – so it is by no means hopeless, **but it is important that couples know how important maternal age is in realistically achieving their dream and so how important it is to get help early particularly if the woman is older**.

In a woman over 45 years old, the chance of spontaneous natural pregnancy is approximately 1%. If the couple do manage to get pregnant, the risk of miscarriage is over 50%. The reason is that virtually all their eggs are genetically abnormal. We occasionally see women who are 43-44 years old and these consultations often prove to be difficult, since the patients have to be informed that the chance of them getting pregnant with their own eggs is very small… not impossible… but pretty remote. But you can only fix something or sort it out if you deal with the truth. Patients often quote famous women having babies well into their 40s and are disheartened to hear our suspicions that many of them have had IVF using donor eggs (eggs donated from much younger women).

So, the message is:

1. Infertility is very common – 1 in 6-7 couples – you are not alone

2. If you are young with a normal AMH, to get pregnant naturally can take time – do not despair.

3. If you can avoid waiting until you are over 35 years old to have children, do so – your fertility significantly reduces and the miscarriage rates go up the older you are.

4. Certainly, if you have been trying for a year or more to conceive (regular unprotected intercourse) and nothing has happened – get medical help. The older you are, the more important this becomes.

5. If there is a family history of Early Menopause (less than 40 years of age), seek medical advice and get tested.

6. If in doubt – get an AMH/FSH and/or an ultrasound scan to ensure that you have good ovarian reserve with a satisfactory reserve of eggs.

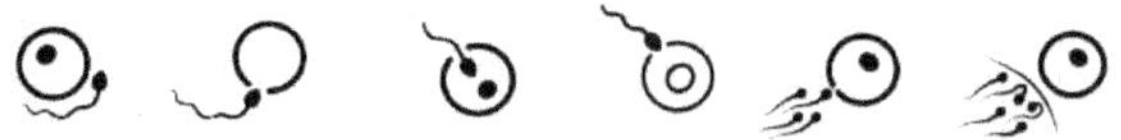

CHAPTER 2

THE FEMALE REPRODUCTIVE SYSTEM (AND HOW IT WORKS)

Introduction

During the course of this chapter, we just want to go through what we normally say/explain to couples in clinic with regard to what happens during a normal menstrual cycle, the timing and frequency of sex that is required and the natural success rates per cycle of trying. Understanding is the key to identifying the possible simple pitfalls as to why you are not managing to get pregnant.

What do I need to get pregnant?

- A normal womb (or uterus) with a healthy endometrium (lining of the womb)
- Open, healthy fallopian tubes
- One or both ovaries that produce eggs
- Normal mobile sperm
- Regular unprotected penetrative sex

A natural cycle – 5 simple steps

There are essentially 5 simple steps in a woman's natural cycle that result either in a pregnancy or menstruation. These are outlined below:

Step 1

Following a period, a hormone called FSH or Follicle Stimulating Hormone is produced by the brain. FSH does what is says on the tin – it stimulates the formation of follicles (a follicle is like a small sac-like structure in the ovary that contains an egg – you will remember we discussed the presence and number of antral follicles in chapter 1). During a natural cycle, one of these follicles (under the influence of FSH) becomes dominant and grows until it reaches about 18-20mm in size, at which point it is ready to release an egg (ovulation).

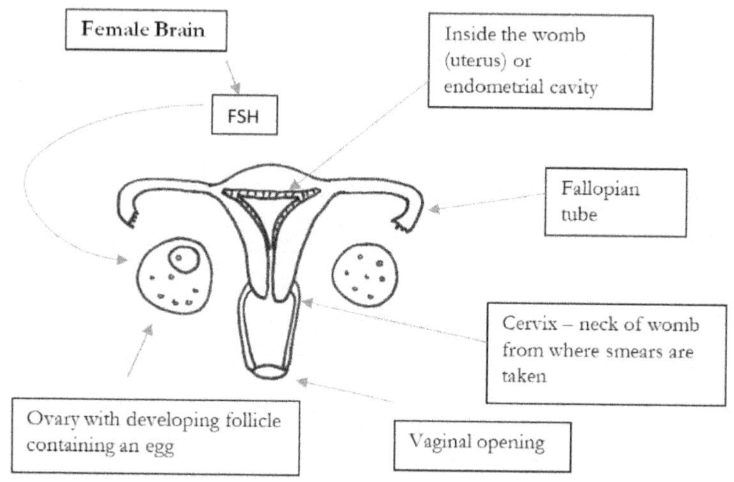

Step 2

Once the dominant follicle reaches 18-20mm in size, it sends a signal to the brain which in response releases another hormone called LH (Luteinising Hormone). It is LH that stimulates ovulation or release of the egg from the ovary and the egg is picked up by the fallopian tube.

Step 3

The couple have sex and millions of sperm are deposited in the vagina from where they swim through the cervix (or neck of the womb), through the uterus and into the tube where they hopefully meet an egg. Just one of these millions of sperm penetrates the egg (fertilisation) to form an embryo. Very occasionally two eggs are produced by the ovaries simultaneously and this results in non- identical twins.

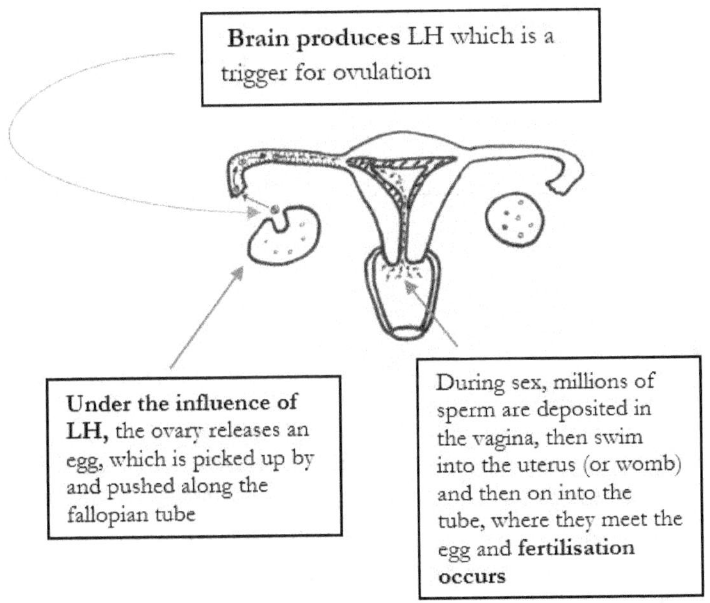

Step 4

The embryo (or fertilised egg) makes its way down the tube into the uterus and implants into the lining of the womb otherwise known as endometrium.

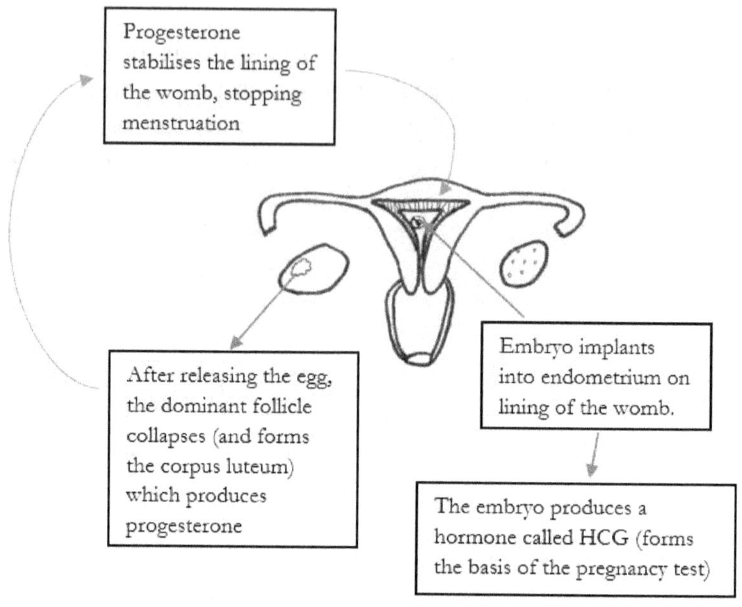

Step 5

The embryo now starts to grow and releases a hormone called HCG (Human chorionic gonadotrophin). This is the hormone that causes a pregnancy test to turn positive. The ovarian follicle, having released its egg, collapses on itself and becomes known as the corpus luteum – it is this that produces progesterone. Progesterone stabilises the endometrium (lining of the womb) preventing menstruation so that the pregnancy continues. The HCG stabilises the corpus luteum which continues to produce progesterone, which continues to stabilise the endometrium, so no period occurs and the pregnancy continues.

If there is no implantation of the embryo, then the pregnancy test is negative (no HCG is produced). If no HCG is produced then the production of progesterone stops, the endometrial lining becomes compromised and a period starts.

If all this works what are the chances of spontaneous pregnancy for every month of trying?

The chance of a woman becoming pregnant per cycle of trying is between **5-25%** depending on the age of the woman. This is not the most efficient of nature's pathways, and particularly since thereafter, the miscarriage rate is in double figures and is again age dependent. Thus if you are a relatively young woman (<35 years old) do not despair if you haven't conceived after 6 months, time is on your side and FURTHER ATTEMPTS should be made. If, however, you are older than 35 years, we would suggest at the very least having an AMH to ensure good ovarian reserve. If the AMH is low, seek help. If you have been trying to get pregnant unsuccessfully for a year or more, seek help whatever your age.

What are the important reproductive hormones that you produce and what do they do?

There are 5 important hormones as follows:

(i) FSH (Follicle Stimulating Hormone) – produced by the brain to stimulate the ovaries to stimulate follicles that contain eggs.

(ii) Oestrogen – a hormone produced by the ovaries which stimulates the endometrium (the lining of the womb) to thicken up ready for implantation of the embryo.

(iii) LH (Luteinising Hormone) – produced by the brain to stimulate release of an egg from the ovarian follicle.

(iv) Progesterone – produced by the collapsed ovarian follicle (corpus luteum) after release of the egg to stabilise the endometrium and stop menstruation.

(v) HCG (Human Chorionic Gonadotrophin) – produced by the implanted embryo and responsible for the positive pregnancy tests. **The purpose of the HCG is to stabilise the corpus luteum which therefore continues to produce progesterone. Since progesterone** stabilises the endometrium you do not have a period and the pregnancy continues.

When trying to get pregnant can you monitor these hormones to improve timing/establish if you are ovulating?

1. Ovulation kits are available from the chemist – these merely measure LH levels in your urine. A raised LH level would indicate ovulation and so aids the timing of intercourse. Clearly if during the course of a menstrual cycle, a woman does not appear to have a LH positive test, she may not be ovulating and therefore should seek help.

2. Another test to determine whether or not ovulation is taking place, is a "Day 21 Progesterone Test", which can be sorted out via your GP. Following ovulation, the collapsed ovarian follicle or corpus luteum produces progesterone. Therefore if your GP does a blood test in the second half of your cycle and the progesterone level is raised – it is likely that you ovulated that month.

The reason that it is called a "Day 21" Progesterone Test is because in the case of a woman with a 28-day cycle, progesterone levels are found to be highest on day 21. A woman will almost always ovulate 14 days before her period and the progesterone levels will be highest 7 days after ovulation – so in a woman with a 28-day cycle, she will ovulate on day 14 and progesterone will be highest on day 21.

It is also worth mentioning that if a woman has 30-day cycles, she is likely to be ovulating on day 16 and therefore progesterone levels will be highest on day 23. Hence, a day 21 progesterone may well be negative in a woman with a 30-day cycle, even if she is ovulating. In

such circumstances ask for a day 23 progesterone for confirmation (See Chapter 4).

3. Pregnancy tests are available from the chemist and they measure HCG levels in your urine that indicate if you are pregnant.

When and how often should you have sex to optimise your chance of getting pregnant?

It is important to remember that **sperm can last up to 6 days in the female genital tract**, and that a released egg can last up to **24** hours. So you do not have to have sex every hour on the hour around the time you ovulate! In fact this can be detrimental to your chances of conception. Remember that the sperm count is at its most potent if ejaculation occurs every 2-3 days. Also remember that ovulation occurs consistently 14 days prior to the start of your period, as long as you have a reasonably regular period. The diagram below indicates best timing for intercourse:

28 day cycle -

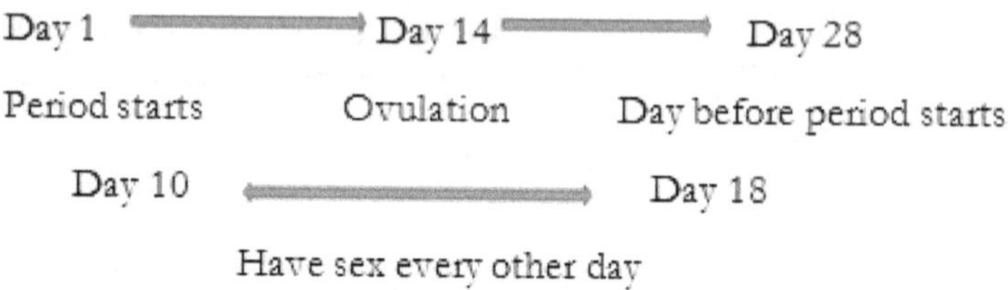

32 day cycle -

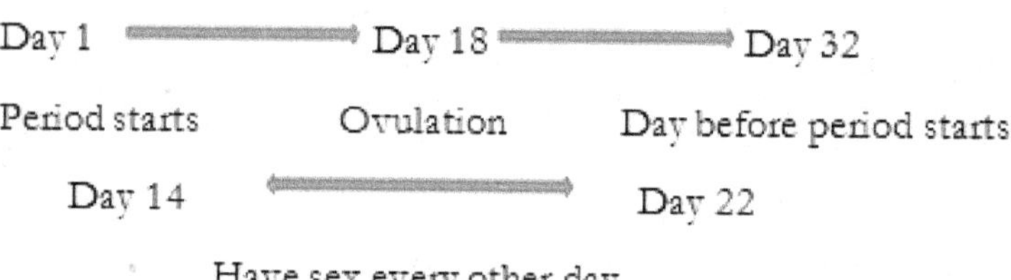

Are there any physical signs that indicate ovulation?

Change in Cervical Mucus – your cervical mucus changes around the time of ovulation. It goes from being relatively thick and scanty to a clearer, more watery consistency, and there is usually more of it.

Basal Body Temperature (BBT) – after ovulation your body temperature rises by about 0.4 degrees. Some women will take their own temperature around the same time every day until a sudden rise, usually mid-cycle, indicates ovulation.

So the message is:

1. In fertility, there are 5 simple steps to how your body works and 5 main hormones of which to be aware.

2. The chance of getting pregnant naturally per month of trying is 5-25% depending on the age of the woman – so do not despair if you are not pregnant after 3-6 months of unprotected sex.

3. If you are older than 35 years and have been trying for 6 months with no luck – check out an AMH test to ensure you have normal ovarian reserve. If it is low… get help.

4. You will ovulate 14 days before you menstruate. So in a woman with a 28-day cycle you will ovulate on day 14, in a woman with a 32-day cycle you will ovulate on day 18 and so on – this is important for timing sex.

5. Sperm last up to 6 days in the female body after sex, so there is usually good overlap and you do not need to have sex every day – it is better to have it every other day.

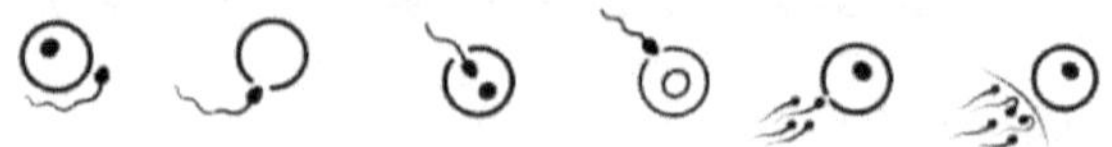

CHAPTER 3

SO, YOU CAN'T GET PREGNANT. WHY NOT?

This chapter details the reasons for the one in six to seven couples in the UK being unable to conceive, and then we will explain what investigations you need and what investigations you should ask for if you have been unable to get pregnant.

First of all – no blame culture

When we see couples coming through the door of the infertility clinic, or indeed these days when we carry out a virtual consultation, it is important to establish an open, honest, and constructive atmosphere in order to move forward. On rare occasions during these consultations, there is what we can only describe as an "an atmosphere". One of the couple looks slightly uncomfortable or even sheepish because "blame" for the couple's inability to have a child has already been decided. The very first thing that needs to be done in such circumstances is to remove such "blame" from the equation. Not only is it unhelpful, but can be destructive within the relationship. The path of conception, pregnancy and birth is not an easy one and the couple need to be mutually loving and supportive of each other to succeed in their quest to have a child. Reference to the problem being "someone's fault" will never help and we would therefore ask you to avoid such judgement, using all your energy positively to achieve your mutual dream.

The approximate rule of thirds

There is usually a rule of thirds with regard to why a couple cannot conceive:

1/3 of the time – problem with the woman.

1/3 of the time – problem with the man.

1/3 of the time – unexplained.

In order to get pregnant a woman must have a uterus with a normal lining of the womb (or endometrium), at least one unblocked fallopian tube; at least one working ovary producing an egg on a regular basis (that usually means regular cycles), a partner with a normal sperm count and unprotected sex at the right time of the month. There is no reason why a woman cannot have a baby with just one ovary, or indeed one open fallopian tube, however, on occasions this may reduce the chances of pregnancy. One third of the time, infertile couples can go through all the investigations outlined below and they are ALL normal. The diagnosis is then one of "UNEXPLAINED INFERTILITY" – these couples generally need help with fertility treatments, particularly if they having been trying to conceive for 18 months with no success.

Reasons for Infertility

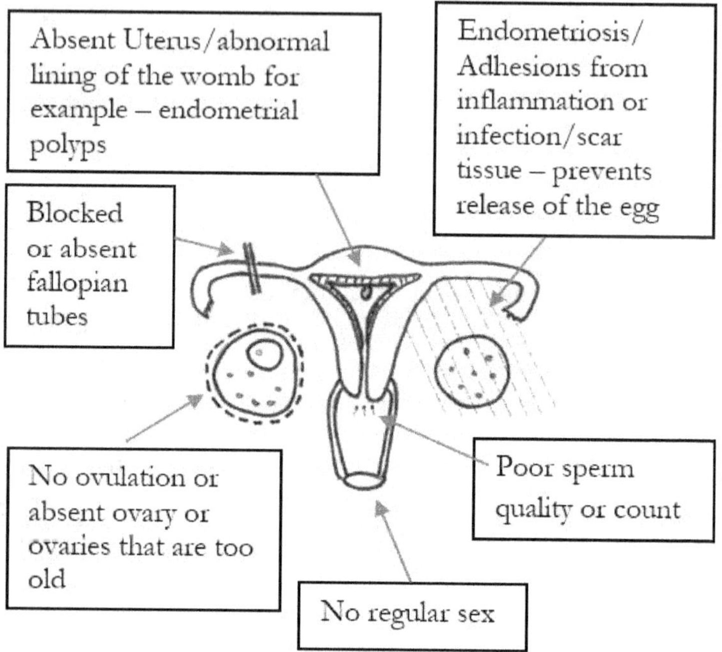

No Uterus/Womb

Evidently if a woman does not have a uterus, she cannot carry a baby. There are a number of reasons for an absent uterus, including having had a previous hysterectomy for all sorts of medical reasons or the fact that the woman was born without a uterus (congenital). This does not necessarily stop a couple having their own child. In fact in the past we have been privileged enough to help couples in whom the women did not have a uterus, have their own biological child. If you still have your own ovaries, it is entirely possible to remove eggs from you using IVF techniques, fertilise your eggs with your partner's sperm and place the resultant embryo into a surrogate (a friend, sister, or altruistic person). They then have your baby for you, much the same as occurred in the hit television series *"Friends"* when *Phoebe* becomes the surrogate for her brother and his wife who end up with triplets. Although this example was fictional, surrogacy is a real and active ongoing treatment option for heterosexual couples when the female partner cannot carry a child or indeed for a same-sex male couple.

Abnormal Lining (endometrium) of the Womb/Polyps/Fibroids

The lining of the womb or endometrium can on occasions be distorted by small- or medium-sized outgrowths called polyps that project into the endometrial cavity. It *may* be that these polyps or outgrowths prevent implantation of the embryo or indeed they may even have a role in miscarriage. Removal of these polyps will help with normal implantation and probably reduce the risk of miscarriage.

On occasions there is scarring of the endometrial lining that can be caused by excessive "curettage" or "scrapping" of the endometrial lining during previous operations such as surgical evacuation following miscarriage or termination of pregnancy. Assessment of the endometrial lining by using a fibre-optic camera or hysteroscope that looks into the endometrial cavity is required and sometimes the damaged endometrial lining can be repaired either surgically or by using high-dose oestrogen.

In addition, it is thought that the existence of fibroids (that occur in at least a third of all women of reproductive age), particularly those fibroids indenting the endometrium (called *submucous* fibroids), may have a role in reducing implantation rates and increasing pregnancy loss.

Blocked or Damaged Fallopian Tubes

This is quite a common phenomenon and one of the commonest reasons for blocked tubes is **PID (Pelvic Inflammatory Disease).** Most of the time this is caused by genital tract infections such as chlamydia (or gonorrhoea). A large percentage of men and women who have had or indeed have chlamydia are asymptomatic (they do not have any symptoms, for example pain or discharge). Hence the infection is not treated and damage continues. Even after treatment with strong antibiotics, scarring may remain and so one or both tubes may be blocked. Obviously if the tubes are blocked the egg and sperm do not meet, then fertilisation cannot occur. If there is damage to the tube the sperm may be able to swim through into the tube and fertilise the egg, but because of tubal damage the fertilised egg (or embryo) never reaches the womb and may implant into the tube itself and an **ectopic pregnancy** results. Hence, in terms of education and awareness the importance of barrier protection to protect against sexually transmitted infection and thereafter *infertility* is hugely relevant. The figures in Table 1 indicate the approximate rates of tubal infertility after infection.

(It is also important to state that pelvic infections such as chlamydia can also cause problems with fertility in men. Genital infection may reduce sperm motility and can also cause abnormality of the sperm DNA, something called *DNA fragmentation*, which will have a significant impact on a man's fertility.)

Table 1. Infection and its relation to tubal infertility:

PID – causing tubal infertility	% of women with severe tubal damage
1st Infection	10-30%
2nd Infection	30-60%
3rd Infection	50-90%

Absent Fallopian Tubes

Fallopian tubes may be absent for a number of reasons. Some

women are born without one or both fallopian tubes (congenital). Others have had surgery to remove one or both fallopian tubes (for example for a past history of ectopic pregnancy – whereby implantation of the pregnancy into the tube occurs, internal bleeding takes place and the tube may need to be surgically removed). It is important to know that if a patient has had a previous ectopic pregnancy, they are at much HIGHER RISK of another ectopic pregnancy in the future. Therefore, in any subsequent pregnancy, an early ultrasound scan (approximately 6 weeks) is indicated to ensure that the pregnancy is sitting in the uterus, not the tube. Early pregnancy units (via your GP) can and should facilitate this.

In addition, if one or both of the fallopian tubes have become diseased or partially blocked because of infection or inflammation, they can become full of fluid and are then called a *"Hydrosalpinx"* (if one tube affected) or if both tubes are affected, *"Hydrosalpinges"* (hydro – meaning water, salpinges – meaning tubes). Invariably, these diseased fallopian tubes do not function well and fertility is impaired. *There is evidence that surgical removal of these "Hydrosalpinges" is beneficial if the woman is to have IVF. Potential toxins can leak from these dilated, fluid-filled tubes into the womb during an IVF cycle, adversely affecting any transferred embryos. Hence removal of the diseased tubes before IVF appears to improve the pregnancy rate.*

Failure to Ovulate

One of the commonest reasons women fail to get pregnant is because they do not ovulate on a regular basis. Probably the commonest reason women do not ovulate is **PCOS (Polycystic Ovarian Syndrome)**. Polycystic ovaries can be seen on a Transvaginal Ultrasound Scan. Women with PCOS usually do not have periods on a regular basis. A woman who has a regular period every 28 to 30 days is likely to be ovulating. However, to test for ovulation a "Day 21" progesterone blood test can be performed – see Chapters 2/4.

If the ovary is absent, either from previous surgery for ovarian cysts or endometriosis, then obviously an egg cannot be produced from that side.

Another reason for not ovulating regularly is ***abnormal thyroid levels*** – this can easily be tested with another blood test known as ***"Thyroid Function Test" (TFTs)*** and treated as required.

A slightly more uncommon reason for women not to ovulate is because of a small growth in the brain called a "prolactinoma" which secretes a hormone called ***prolactin*** – a simple blood test can be done to ensure that this is normal.

Finally, **the age of the eggs is a big deal.** If you are in your 20s, your chance of conception is 20-25% per month of trying. If you are in your 40s, your chance of conception is about 5% per month of trying.

No Regular Sex

Some couples present to a fertility clinic after trying unsuccessfully to conceive for 12 to 18 months, and when questioned it becomes apparent that they live separate lives – for example, she lives in London and he lives in Cardiff. When they do see each other, they may have intercourse, but often it is poorly timed with the woman's ovulation and infrequent. It is worth remembering that if all investigations are normal and REGULAR intercourse takes place, the average chance of conception per month of trying, is maximally 25% (age dependent). So, if the sex that a couple are having is infrequent and not at the right time, it is likely to take a good deal longer for them to achieve a pregnancy.

Male Factors

Abnormal sperm count, motility (how well the sperm move), and abnormal sperm appearance/structure are not uncommon in couples seeking help. Male factor problems are responsible for the infertility in about a third of the cases seen. It is treatable with assisted reproduction techniques (IUI, IVF and ICSI) which will be described in future chapters. In addition, there are other problems encountered by the male partner which can affect fertility including impotence or the inability to have an erection. Please see Chapter 13 (All Things to do with Sperm, Male Infertility and the Use of Donor Sperm).

Endometriosis/Adhesions

Another common reason for subfertility is the presence of adhesions and "endometriosis". Endometriosis in its simplest terms is when deposits of the lining of your womb (endometrium) grow outside the womb. Every month the lining of the womb grows and bleeds, resulting in a period. If you have endometriosis, the endometrial deposits outside the womb and commonly in the pelvis also grow and bleed. The blood produced in the pelvis is an irritant and inflammation occurs adjacent to the tubes and ovaries, causing scarring/adhesions. Adhesions can be described as fibrous strands of glue-like substance that can pull and fuse adjacent tissues. This may result in distortion of the fallopian tubes and ovaries with subsequent infertility.

Ovarian Endometriosis – as well as causing problems with the tubes, endometriosis can destroy ovarian tissue. "Chocolate cysts" can form in the ovaries. Endometriotic deposits on the ovary bleed at the same time as you menstruate and form pockets of blood within the ovaries. Old blood resembles chocolate – hence the descriptive term "chocolate cysts". In this way endometriosis can destroy ovarian tissue and interfere with ovulation, possibly resulting in problems conceiving.

It is thought that endometriosis may be present in approximately 20-65% of women with infertility, but equally lots of women with endometriosis are able to conceive spontaneously. It can be present in very mild to very severe forms. Some women who have endometriosis never have any symptoms, have children and never know they have the disease. Others present to their doctors with severe symptoms of pelvic pain, painful periods, and pain when they have sex. The gold standard to investigate endometriosis is a "Laparoscopy". This is a camera through the umbilicus (belly button) when the patient is asleep with a general anaesthetic. Endometriosis can then be viewed and treated surgically by either excision or ablation (essentially burning it off) or it can be treated medically. Please see Chapter 12 on Endometriosis.

Unexplained Infertility

So what happens if everything is normal? The woman's uterus and endometrial lining is normal AND the woman is ovulating regularly AND the fallopian tubes are open AND the semen analysis is normal AND the couple are having regular intercourse at the right time. If no pregnancy has occurred after 12 to 18 months the diagnosis is of **_Unexplained Infertility. In other words, the medical profession does not know why you are not getting pregnant!_** This will usually mean that you will benefit from either IUI (Intrauterine Insemination) or IVF. **_Please do not despair – many couples with Unexplained Infertility manage to have a child following IUI or IVF treatment._**

So, the message is:

1. If you have been trying to conceive unsuccessfully after having regular intercourse for 12 to 18 months – seek help and referral for proper investigation. If you are older than 35 years, an AMH blood test to ensure a normal ovarian reserve is reassuring prior to trying for 12-18 months.

2. The reasons couples cannot conceive are approximately divided into thirds. A third of the time there is a problem with the woman, a third of the time there is a problem with the man, but a third of the time all the investigations are normal (unexplained subfertility).

3. Pelvic infection can cause infertility - take care if you are going to have casual sex, and use a condom to protect yourself – after one attack of chlamydia, up to 30% of the time your tubes will become diseased and blocked, rendering you more likely to have an ectopic pregnancy or infertile.

4. If you think you (him or her) have PID (Pelvic Inflammatory Disease) go to your nearest Genitourinary Medicine Clinic (GUM clinic) present in most NHS hospitals and get checked. The earlier you treat PID, the better.

5. If you are worried you have endometriosis, the most accurate way of knowing if you really have it is to do a laparoscopy – ask your GP for referral.

6. Do not wait too long to have your children – when you are 20 years old, your chance of pregnancy is 20-25% per month of trying to conceive. When you are 40 years old, your chance of pregnancy is 5% per month of trying to conceive.

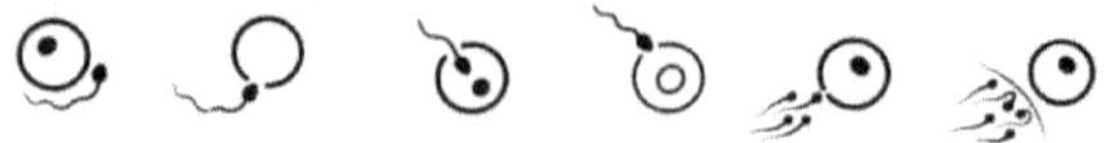

CHAPTER 4

WHAT INVESTIGATIONS DO YOU NEED?

Having established why infertility occurs, what do you do next and what investigations are appropriate and can be arranged by your GP or Infertility Specialist?

In the first instance, an appointment with your GP is appropriate and there are a few investigations that hopefully they will be able to sort out for you. Certainly, if you have been trying to conceive for over a year with no success, it seems reasonable to request a referral to a gynaecologist (at your local hospital), who should be able to complete any further investigations. If the results of those investigations show that the couple need a fertility treatment like IVF for example, then onward referral to a tertiary Fertility Clinic is required – this can be facilitated both for advice and indeed any treatment that might be indicated. All this takes time, and many patients will bypass this pathway and seek help by going to a private Fertility Clinic.

It is important to know, however, at least for patients living in the UK, that they are entitled to investigation and treatment on the NHS, if that couple have no children together and have been unable to conceive despite trying for 12-18 months.

FOR HER – What basic investigations do I need?

Transvaginal ultrasound scan (TVUS)

A good basic investigation for the woman is to have an ultrasound scan of the pelvis. As the name suggests, this is done "trans-vaginally" by a small probe that goes into the vagina. The uterus, the endometrial lining, and the ovaries can be viewed and abnormalities detected. This scan can identify:

1. Fibroids – benign growths in the wall of the womb that can affect fertility.

2. Endometrial polyps – small growths in the endometrial lining of the womb that can prevent implantation and increase the risk of miscarriage.

3. Ovarian cysts/possibly endometriosis of the ovaries ("endometriomas")/polycystic ovaries (associated with lack of ovulation and therefore potential difficulty in achieving conception)

4. The AFC – the Antral Follicle Count (the number of small follicles or sac-like structures within the ovary) that indicate a patient's ovarian or egg reserve.

5. The fallopian tubes cannot be seen with ultrasound scan because they are too small. If, however, a tube is damaged and full of fluid (known as a hydrosalpinx), it becomes visible on ultrasound.

Are you ovulating? To see whether you are ovulating you can have a "Day 21 Progesterone Test" with your doctor.

This is a simple test that measures the hormone progesterone and has previously been discussed in Chapter 2. Progesterone is released by the ovary after ovulation occurs, and can be measured with a blood test. If the blood test shows a certain increased level, it is likely that the patient has ovulated. The timing of the blood test during your cycle depends on the length of your cycle. The golden rule is that you will almost always ovulate 14 days before you have a period, and if you have ovulated the progesterone level will be highest 7 days after that. So, in a 28-day cycle have your progesterone level measured on day 21 (21 days after the start of your period). In a 30-day cycle, have your progesterone measured on day 23 (23 days after the start of your period). Finally in a 32-day cycle, have your progesterone measured on day 25 (25 days after the start of your period). **Menstrual cycles that last longer than 35 days, are often irregular and women are less likely to be ovulating on a regular basis.** The diagrams below illustrate the timing of the progesterone blood test:

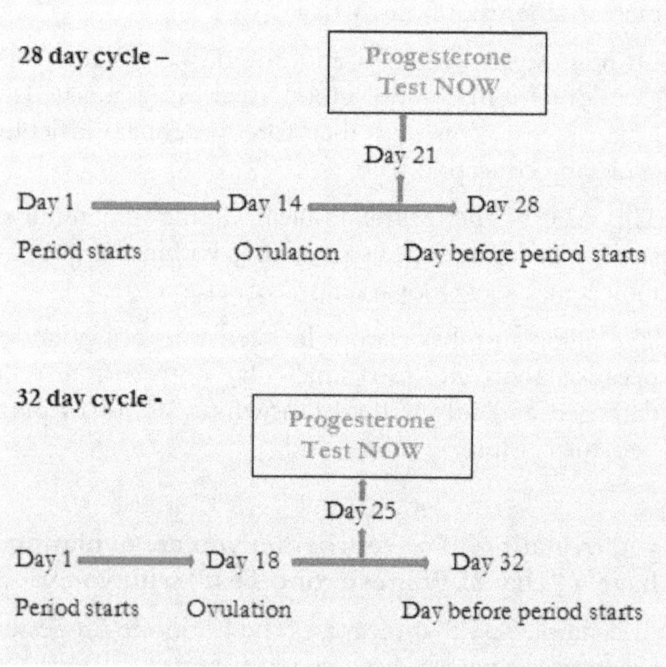

If these tests show that you are not ovulating, you will need to have further blood tests including a Thyroid Function Test (TFT) and Serum Prolactin carried out. If

your thyroid gland in your neck is producing too much or too little of the hormone thyroxine, it can affect whether you ovulate on a regular basis. Also, if your brain produces too much prolactin, your ability to ovulate is affected. Therefore, TFTs and Prolactin are often carried out routinely as an investigation for the female partner.

Are you ovulating? An alternate method you can use at home to see whether you are ovulating is to test your urine with the "LH Hormone Ovulation test".

This is a simple kit that you can buy from your local chemist. Essentially when you think you are due to ovulate (instructions are given with the kit), you pee onto a stick. This is then plugged into a small monitor that reads whether you have LH (luteinising hormone) in your urine. You will remember that LH is the signal from the brain for the ovary to release its egg. So if higher levels of LH are detected in the urine it is likely that you are soon to ovulate and sexual intercourse can be timed to maximise your chance of pregnancy. You will normally ovulate 34-36 hours after the LH "surge". One word of caution – this test may not work so well with women who have polycystic ovaries because they may have elevated levels of LH throughout the cycle.

How many eggs have I got left? There are 3 tests that can indicate a patient' ovarian reserve:

1. **AMH (Anti Mullerian Hormone)** is a simple blood test that can be taken at any time of the month within a woman's cycle. It gives information about how many eggs are left in the ovaries of the individual woman having the test. If the AMH is low, then there are fewer eggs left in the ovaries, menopause is closer and timely treatment to aid conception is required with likely higher doses of medication to stimulate the ovaries to produce eggs. Conversely, if the AMH is normal or higher, then

more eggs are left in the ovaries and menopause is further away. This knowledge allows the individual to be slightly more relaxed. This test is usually only done in fertility clinic settings and not available at the GPs.

2. **FSH** is a simple blood test done in the first 2-4 days of the menstrual cycle and can be done at the GP's surgery. If the FSH is high, it can indicate a poorer ovarian reserve and limited time to conceive.

3. **AFC (Antral Follicle Count)** – as discussed with a transvaginal ultrasound scan.

If you are going to see the GP they may carry out the following tests:

Day 2-4 FSH / LH / Serum Prolactin / Thyroid Function Tests / Day 21 Progesterone / Ultrasound scan of the pelvis

If you are seen by a gynaecologist, they may carry out hospital-based investigations:

An HSG – to see if your tubes are open

A Hysteroscopy – to look inside your womb

A Laparoscopy – to look inside your tummy

These are explained later in the chapter.

If you are seen in a Fertility Clinic, they will usually ask for:

An AMH and it is here that treatments such as IVF are carried out

Are your tubes blocked? To see whether your tubes are blocked you will need a Hysterosalpingogram (HSG).

This is usually done in an X-ray department of your local

hospital. You do not need an anaesthetic. During an HSG, a small soft tube or catheter is placed into the neck of the womb or cervix. Dye is injected into the womb and if the tubes are open, the dye will spill out of the ends of the tubes and into your tummy. An X-ray of the pelvis is taken and will show an outline of the uterus, tubes, and the dye spilling out into your tummy. You then know that your fallopian tubes are open.

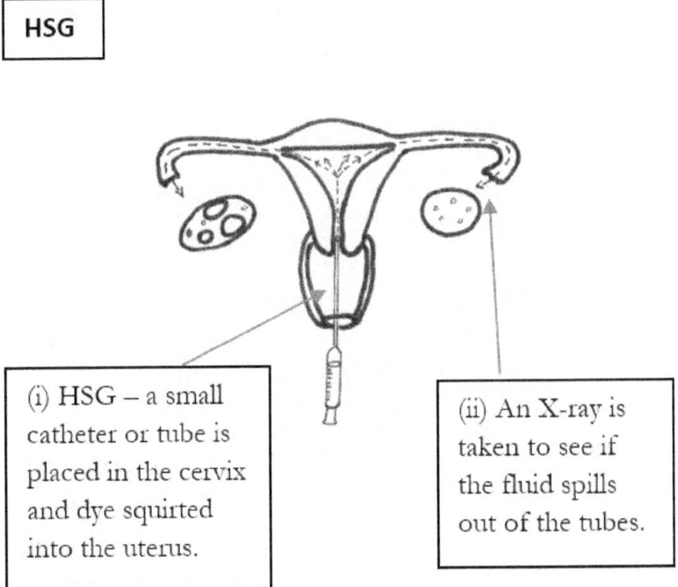

(i) HSG – a small catheter or tube is placed in the cervix and dye squirted into the uterus.

(ii) An X-ray is taken to see if the fluid spills out of the tubes.

Another test to check the fallopian tubes that you may be offered is the **"HyCoSy"** test or **Hysterosalpingo-Contrast-Sonography**. Put simply, this is very similar to the HSG test except that it uses ultrasound scanning instead of X-rays. Like an HSG, it is done without the need for any anaesthetic (patients may get some mild to moderate cramping in the pelvis). During a HyCoSy, a small, thin tube is placed into the womb and a substance that shows up on ultrasound scanning is injected. This fills the womb and the fallopian tubes so that tubal patency (open tubes) can be identified when an ultrasound scan is carried out.

Is the lining of your womb normal? To see whether the lining of your womb (endometrium) is normal, the 'gold standard' investigation is a hysteroscopy.

As already explained, a transvaginal ultrasound scan (TVUS) will often show up endometrial polyps or the possibility of "damaged" endometrium. If there is any doubt, direct viewing of the endometrium can be achieved with hysteroscopy. Having a hysteroscopy is essentially introducing a "fibre-optic camera" on the end of a metal rod into the womb to look at the endometrial cavity and occasionally to take a biopsy from it. Sometimes the lining of the womb can be distorted by having small growths called polyps or sub-mucous fibroids. These can stop the implantation of the embryo into the lining of the womb and so stop you getting pregnant. Alternatively, they may also cause miscarriage. These polyps or sub-mucous fibroids can often be removed at the time of the hysteroscopy.

We have seen a number of patients who have been unable to have a baby and following hysteroscopy with identification and subsequent removal of these polyps, successful pregnancies have ensued.

In addition, sometimes other abnormalities of the inside of the uterus / endometrium are seen that are either congenital – for example, a division or septum inside the womb or indeed scar tissue from previous surgery. To diagnose these abnormalities with the potential for discussion for ongoing treatment is facilitated by hysteroscopy.

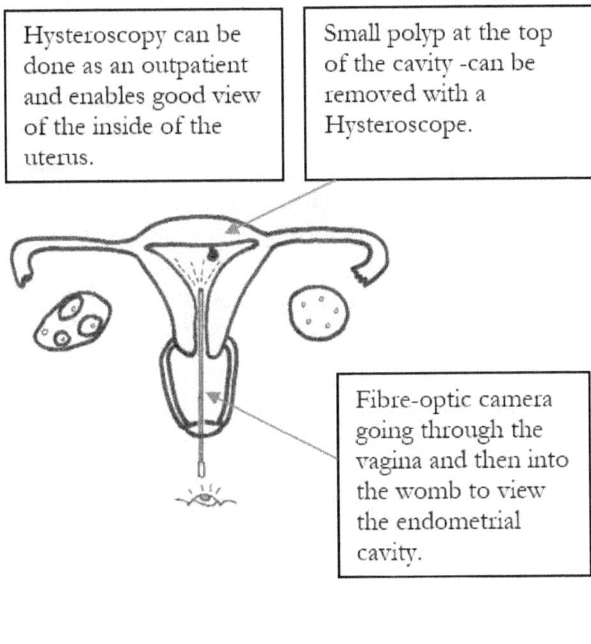

Is your pelvis normal, do you have Endometriosis? If there is a suspicion of endometriosis, you may be referred to have a laparoscopy

During laparoscopy, which is the same as "keyhole" surgery, a fibre-optic camera is placed through the tummy button to directly look into the pelvis. Any Endometriosis or scar tissue can be identified and treated. Also the tubes can be checked to see if they are blocked by squirting blue dye through the cervix in much the same manner as the HSG. If there are no blockages, dye is seen coming out of the ends of the tubes and spilling into your tummy. This procedure needs to be done under a general anaesthetic.

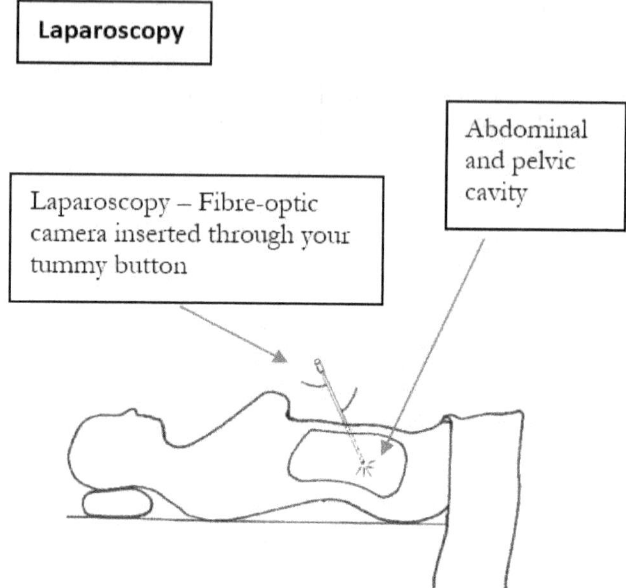

It is important to state that the request for an investigation should be influenced by a person's previous medical history which needs to be taken in detail prior to ordering any tests. Certainly, some of the investigations listed above are not necessary for all women. For example, if the scan of the pelvis is normal and shows a normal endometrial lining, normal uterus and normal ovaries, that woman does NOT necessarily need a laparoscopy or indeed hysteroscopy.

For men, again it is important to take a full clinical history that might give a lead as to the possibility of male factor infertility. For example, a history of using anabolic steroids can cause major problems with male fertility and sometimes you have the potential diagnosis before you have done the tests. For the male partner it is also important to know that there are no problems with impotence or indeed ejaculation. Thereafter, the main and single most important test is the Semen Analysis:

FOR HIM – What Investigations do I need?

THERE IS ONE BASIC INVESTIGATION FOR THE MALE PARTNER

Is your Sperm Sample Normal? Semen Analysis Test

To see whether your sperm is normal you need to have a "Semen Analysis" test. The Semen Analysis test is a microscopic examination of the male ejaculate. Semen is the fluid in which the sperm swim. The specimen should be produced by masturbation into a dry, clean container. This should be examined in the laboratory ideally within 30 minutes of ejaculation. No sex or masturbation should have taken place for **2-5** days before the sample is produced. Most fertility units provide a "Semen-analysis Room" (ideally a clean, quiet, comfortable and private room), where the male partner produces his sample. Occasionally the couple will go into the room together where she can provide encouragement to his efforts. If the sample is produced on site the laboratory can examine the sample almost immediately, promoting an accurate result. Sometimes it is difficult for the male partner to provide a sample "on demand" within a fertility unit and he may have to produce a sample at home and bring it in. Within most of these rooms, the unit provide appropriate pictorial literature to help with the production of a sample.

Table A. World Health Organisation (2010) – normal values for Semen Samples:

Volume per ejaculate	1.5ml
Concentration	15 million sperm/ml
Progressive Motility	32%
Normal Forms	> or = 4%

What does Table A. mean?

(a) The first value (volume of the ejaculate) is reasonably self-explanatory – and refers to how much seminal fluid is produced following ejaculation. You need at least 1.5ml of ejaculate to be normal – some men produce a great deal more than this which is still normal, others less than this which is by the above criteria abnormal and may be the reason for impaired fertility.

(b) The second value (concentration) refers to the concentration of the sperm within the sample. Again some men have concentrations of sperm up to and beyond 50 million sperm for every ml of ejaculate, but as long as you have at least 15 million sperm for every ml of seminal fluid produced, you are within the normal range. It can be seen that if you produce 1.5ml of ejaculate with a concentration of 15 million per ml, the total number of sperm in the sample will be 22.5 million.

(c) The third value – Progressive Motility – refers to the active *forward* movement of the sperm that can be seen. You may have 100% motility of sperm but if they are all swimming around and around and going nowhere fast, it isn't much good. There has to be progressive forward movement and if a third of your sperm are doing this, you are normal.

(d) Finally, Morphology – this refers to what the sperm look like. If they look abnormal or their structure is not right then they have abnormal *Morphology*. Interestingly enough you only need a very small proportion of the sperm to look normal (4% as per the above table), for the sample to be normal.

It is likely that the concentration and progressive motility are the most important values in predicting the chance of pregnancy for either normal sexual intercourse or insemination of the sperm higher into the womb (IUI – intrauterine insemination). Certainly when the concentration is less than 10 million per ml or the progressive motility is less than 20%, normal sexual intercourse or even IUI is unlikely to work and IVF may be a better option. IVF techniques can achieve pregnancy with markedly low sperm counts.

However, it is important to point out that you only need one good sperm in the right place for conception to take place and even if the sperm count is low – although unlikely, it is not impossible for pregnancy to still occur following normal intercourse.

For further reading on Male Infertility – please see Chapter 13 – All things to do with the Sperm, Male Infertility and the use of Donor Sperm.

So, the message is:

1. Basic investigations include a Transvaginal Ultrasound Scan (TVUS) of the pelvis, mid-luteal progesterone (Day 21 in case of a 28-day cycle) to check if you are ovulating, HSG to check tubal patency, and semen analysis.

2. If you are not ovulating check TFTs (Thyroid Function Tests) and prolactin, abnormalities of which can prevent ovulation.

3. If there is a suggestion of endometrial polyps on TVUS have a hysteroscopy.

4. If there is a suspicion of endometriosis consider a laparoscopy.

5. If you have been trying to conceive for 12 to 18 months with no success – ask for ongoing referral.

6. Especially if you are nearing 35 years of age, consider an AMH blood test to check your ovarian reserve.

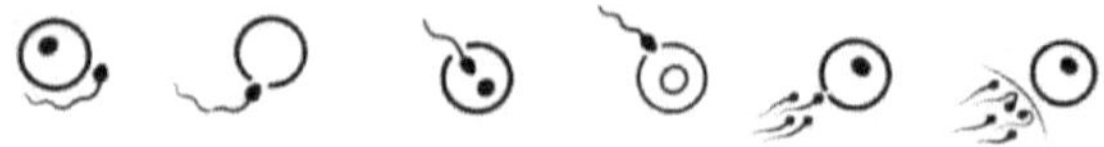

CHAPTER 5

WHAT FERTILITY TREATMENTS ARE AVAILABLE AND WHICH ONE DO YOU NEED?

What fertility treatments are available?

There are essentially 4 main differing treatments that can be used in infertility clinics to help infertile couples to achieve the dream of having a baby of their own. Depending on each individual or couple's requirements, there will necessarily be variation on how each treatment is carried out. In the event of there being no sperm or eggs available, donor eggs or donor sperm, or sometimes both can be employed. If an individual or couple do not have a uterus or are unable to carry their own child, for example in the case of a woman who has had a hysterectomy or in a same-sex male couple, then a surrogate uterus is also required.

In addition, if the semen analysis shows that there are no sperm (for example in the case of a man who has had a vasectomy in the past), then a ***surgical*** sperm retrieval can obtain enough sperm for a treatment to achieve pregnancy for that couple.

Four main treatments available are:

1. **Ovulation Induction with *Clomid* or *Letrozole* (with ultrasound monitoring)**

2.   **IUI (Intrauterine Insemination)**

3.   **IVF (In Vitro Fertilisation)**

4.   **ICSI (Intracytoplasmic Sperm Injection)**

Use of donor eggs or donor sperm – it is important to remember if the couple's own sperm or eggs are deficient or absent, then donor sperm or eggs can be used. Likewise, the use of a surrogate uterus is also possible.

Having established the reasons for infertility, what treatment do you need?

Not Ovulating – *Clomid/Letrozole*/IUI/IVF

Damaged or Absent Tubes – IVF/ICSI

Unexplained Infertility – IUI/IVF/ICSI

Poor Sperm Count – ICSI

No Sperm (post-vasectomy) – Surgical sperm retrieval and ICSI or use of donor sperm

Severe Endometriosis – IUI/IVF/ICSI

Same-sex Female Couple – Donor sperm with IUI (D-IUI)/Donor sperm with IVF (D-IVF)

Same-sex Male Couple – Donor eggs fertilised in an IVF cycle, then embryo transfer into a surrogate OR an IUI cycle directly into a surrogate

Absent Womb – IVF/ICSI with a surrogate female

Advanced Reproductive Age/Absent Ovaries – IVF with donor eggs

In the following chapters we will briefly describe each treatment in turn and the reasons behind choosing it.

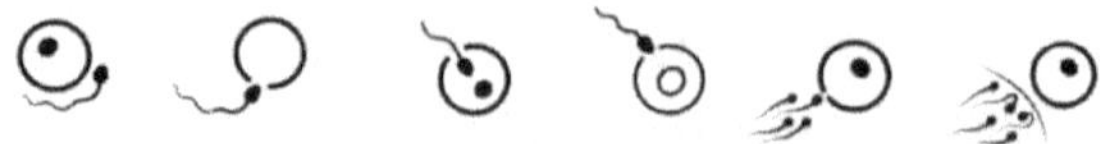

CHAPTER 5A

NOT OVULATING – CLOMID/LETROZOLE WITH FOLLICLE TRACKING

What is *Clomid?*

Clomid is a medication in the form of a tablet. It comes in 50mg, 100mg, or 150mg strengths. For women who are not ovulating, particularly those with established PCOS, *Clomid* can be used to achieve ovulation and hence pregnancy. *Clomid* works by encouraging the human brain to produce a surge of FSH (Follicle Stimulating Hormone). FSH in turn does what it says on the tin – it stimulates the ovaries to develop follicles which have eggs in them, thereby hopefully encouraging ovulation.

How and when do I take *Clomid?*

Day 1 of a woman's cycle is when she starts her period. One tablet of *Clomid* 50mg is taken on a daily basis starting on **day 2-5** and continuing to **day 6-9** (5 days in total during that cycle). This will usually result in a woman ovulating around day 14, hence giving her a 28-day cycle.

***Clomid* is taken for 5 days (Starting between day 2 and day 5 of the cycle)**

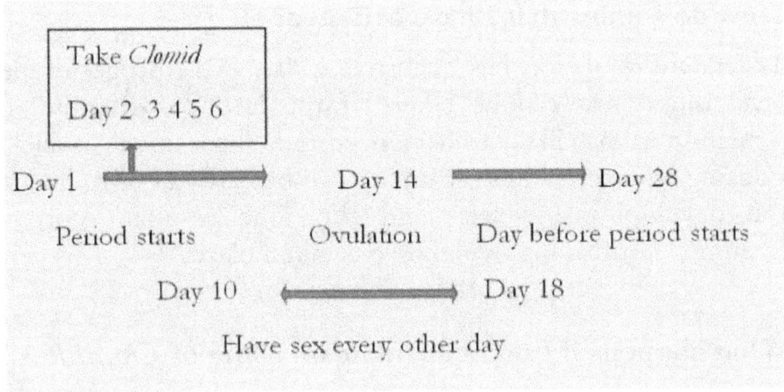

How is the growth of the follicles monitored?

The short answer is with regular ultrasound scans of the pelvis. During a cycle when *Clomid* is used, a series of ultrasound scans are carried out to ensure growth and monitoring of the ovarian follicles. Once a follicle has reached 18-20mm diameter in size, it is likely to ovulate and the couple are advised to have sex every other day to maximise their chance of pregnancy. The first ultrasound scan is usually carried out between day 9 and day 12 of your cycle and then repeated until the follicle(s) reach 18mm. At this point ovulation is likely to occur naturally or a trigger shot injection (*Ovitrelle or Gonasi*) can be used as described below.

How can I better time ovulation?

Once the ovarian follicle(s) have reached 18-20mm (as noted on ultrasound scanning) in size they are mature. At that point, it is possible to induce ovulation with an injection of a hormone akin to LH (it is called *Ovitrelle or Gonasi*). This injection will stimulate ovulation 34-36 hours after it is injected – and so timing of sex can be more precise.

How do I know that I have ovulated?

To ensure ovulation has occurred, a "Day 21" progesterone level blood test can be taken. If the level is >30mmol/l, ovulation is 95% likely to have occurred. Alternatively, follicle tracking with ultrasound scanning can be carried out to image the developing follicle(s) and then the resultant corpus luteum(s) confirming ovulation has taken place.

What happens if I do not ovulate on 50mg of *Clomid*?

If ovulation has not occurred, then the dose of *Clomid* is increased to 100mg during the course of the next cycle. There is probably no advantage in increasing the dose beyond 100mg, although some clinicians will go as high as 150mg.

Generally, it is advised to have no more than 6 months of treatment with *Clomid*. If pregnancy has not been achieved by then, a different treatment mode should be considered.

What are the risks of taking *Clomid*?

The risks of taking *Clomid* include:

1. *Clomid* increases the risk of multiple pregnancy (twins ~5-12%, triplets ~1%). Although we have known some patients who welcome this, it actually means a great deal more risk for that pregnancy, from increased miscarriage risk to a higher incidence of babies being born prematurely – all of which can end in heartache.

2. *Clomid* can cause cystic change of the ovaries.

3. About 10% of women will experience hot flushes. Some may experience visual disturbance which then means it should be stopped.

4. There is a small but serious risk of Ovarian Hyper-stimulation Syndrome (OHSS) which will be explained

later in the book.

5.   One fact that many couples are unaware of is that *Clomid* can cause thinning of lining of the womb (which can be noted with ultrasound scanning) and thickening of cervical mucus (due to its anti-oestrogenic activity). In cases like this, alternative medication such as *Letrozole* (see below) can be used.

It is important to remember that if you are already ovulating, the use of *Clomid* may boost the number of follicles produced by the ovaries, but because of its potential negative effect on the endometrium, pregnancy rates may actually be lower. **So, if you are already ovulating *Clomid* will NOT improve your chance of pregnancy.**

We always insist on the use of ultrasound tracking when *Clomid* is used. This means we can identify the number of follicles and therefore potential eggs and then give advice on the risk of multiple pregnancy, development of ovarian cysts and monitor for OHSS. It also means we can advise on the timing of intercourse and potentially prescribe a 'trigger' shot of LH to induce ovulation (as previously described). Finally, ultrasound scanning gives an assessment of the endometrial lining to ensure that it has not been affected and become thin and unreceptive.

What happens if I do not get a period so cannot start the *Clomid* on day 2?

If you are not having any periods, it is difficult to start Clomid on day 2 of a cycle because you haven't had a monthly cycle! The answer is to use progesterone to induce a bleed and go from there. So, if you have not had a period for 2 months or longer, then check a pregnancy test to make sure that you are not pregnant. If this is negative, then start a progesterone tablet, such as *Norethisterone* (5mg) three times daily for 5 days. You will remember that progesterone stabilises the lining of the womb (endometrium) so that when it is stopped after 5 days, the endometrium is destabilised and menstruation starts. Count this as day 1, then the following day (day 2) start *Clomid*.

So, what are the success rates with *Clomid*?

About 70% of the time, *Clomid* helps non-ovulatory women to produce an egg and if all else is normal with the couple, then **up to** 50% of couples will have achieved pregnancy within 6 months.

What are the alternative medications for *Clomid*?

Letrozole tablets

Although it is not licenced in UK for ovulation induction, many fertility clinics in the UK use *Letrozole* and actually prefer it to *Clomid*. Indeed, it is often used in preference to *Clomid* in many countries. Again it works by increasing the FSH level and thus the number of developing follicles. Like *Clomid, Letrozole* is taken for 5 days starting at the beginning of the cycle on day 2-5. The initial dose is usually 2.5mg that can be increased to 5mg and then to 7.5mg depending on a woman's response as monitored by ultrasound scans.

There is evidence that the use of *Letrozole* gives a higher pregnancy rate when compared to *Clomid* and unlike *Clomid*, it does not affect the endometrial lining or cervical mucus. In addition, it appears to be associated with a lower risk of multiple pregnancy. Hence its favoured use in many fertility institutions worldwide.

Gonadotrophin injections (FSH equivalent)

Gonadotrophin injections (or injections of Follicle Stimulating Hormone – FSH) are the same hormonal injections used in IVF cycles to stimulate growth of follicles. Much lower doses are administered in ovulation induction cycles, to ensure the development of just one or two follicles. It is very important to monitor these cycles closely with ultrasound scans due to increased risk of hyper-stimulation and multiple pregnancy.

So, the message is:

1. If investigations have revealed that you are not ovulating on a regular basis, treatment with *Clomid* is a relatively simple and inexpensive first-line treatment.

2. *Clomid* does *not* improve your chances of pregnancy if you are already ovulating on a regular basis.

3. *Letrozole*, although unlicensed in the UK, is a very good alternative to *Clomid* and in fact many fertility units prefer it to *Clomid*.

4. All treatments with *Clomid, Letrozole* or Gonadotrophins must be monitored with ultrasound.

5. The main risks of these treatments for ovulation induction are those of twin pregnancy, the development of ovarian cysts and hyper-stimulation.

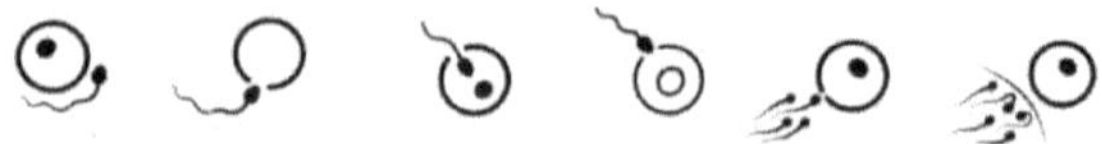

CHAPTER 5B

IUI (INTRA UTERINE INSEMINATION)

What is IUI?

Intra uterine insemination is exactly that – inseminating the woman with her partner's/donor's sperm into her womb to coincide with the time that she is ovulating. This can be done either during a natural cycle or during a medicated cycle when drugs are given to enhance the production of eggs. Ultrasound tracking of the ovarian follicles is carried out prior to the IUI to ensure ovulation is about to take place.

IUI can be used in patients with PCOS who are not ovulating regularly, in patients with unexplained infertility, in patients with endometriosis who cannot get pregnant naturally. It can be used **with donor sperm** in both same-sex couples, or indeed in heterosexual couples in whom the partner's sperm is defective or suboptimal. Finally, it can be used with a surrogate in same-sex male couples.

Reasons for treatment with IUI

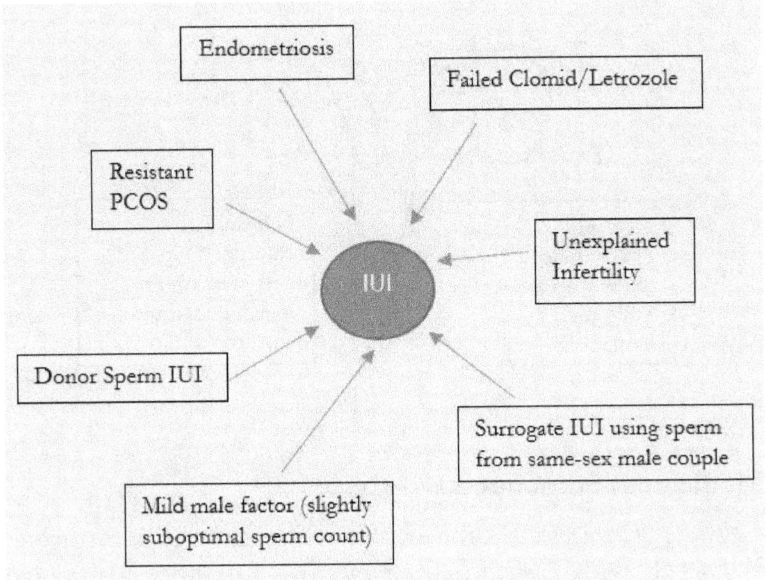

Natural IUI Cycle

Following the start of her period, the woman has a baseline scan to ensure the endometrial lining and ovaries are normal. **A tracking scan is done usually around day 10 to ensure development of dominant follicle.** In a woman with a 28-day cycle, IUI is carried out between day 12 and day 16. A urine or blood test (looking for the rise in LH, which is the trigger for ovulation) is used to determine when ovulation is likely to take place and the partner's/donor's sperm is collected, prepared, and then injected into the womb some 36 hours after the positive LH test (to coincide with ovulation). A pregnancy test is then carried out about 16 days later.

Prior to a natural cycle IUI, the woman should have been tested to ensure that she has open fallopian tubes (with an HSG), has a regular cycle and is ovulating, and that the sperm is adequate after it has been washed down and prepared.

Natural IUI – need open tubes, regular cycles

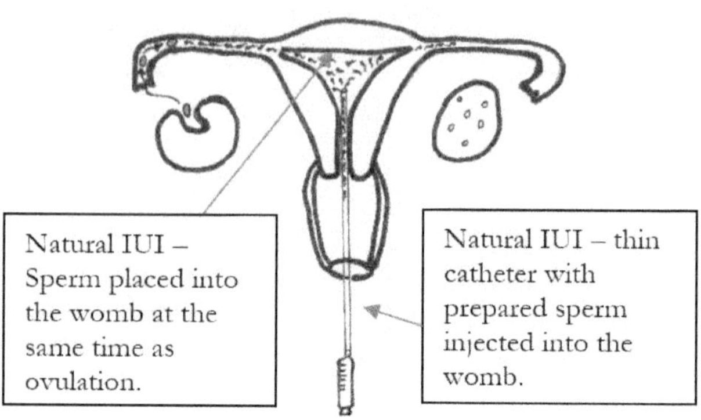

Medicated/Stimulated IUI Cycle

Clomid / Letrozole - Some clinics will carry out a medicated IUI Cycle with *Clomid* or *Letrozole* as a first line to stimulate the ovaries. They will monitor the growth of follicle(s) with ultrasound scans, and when the follicle(s) reach 18-20mm, ovulation can be induced with *Ovitrelle* (or *Gonasi* or *Pregnyl*). Thereafter, 36 hours later they will carry out the insemination.

Gonadotrophins – Follicle Stimulating Hormone (FSH) or its equivalent is also frequently used in medicated IUI cycles thus: Following the start of her period, a baseline scan is carried out to ensure the endometrial lining and ovaries are normal. The woman then starts a small daily injection of a drug that closes down her own hormones (see below re: GnRHa/*Suprecur*). A second daily drug, a gonadotrophin (FSH – Follicle Stimulating Hormone), is then given to stimulate the ovaries to produce follicles containing eggs. Regular scans are then carried out to monitor the growth of the developing follicles. When the follicles reach 18-20mm in size they are thought to be ready to ovulate. At that point, a final injection is given (***Ovitrelle*, Gonasi, Pregnyl**) that causes ovulation, and 36 hours later the IUI is carried out.

In contrast to the natural cycle, there may well be more than 1 follicle produced. Most clinics will proceed with the insemination if there are 2 or 3 mature follicles (with 2 or 3 possible eggs) present. However, ovulation of more than 3 follicles with the insemination of millions of sperm is probably not a good idea since the possibility of triplets or quads then goes right up. If too many follicles are produced, it is possible to continue with the insemination if a "Follicle Reduction" is carried out. This is very similar to a transvaginal egg collection carried out with IVF (see below) and entails draining unwanted follicles via a needle placed through the vagina under ultrasound guidance to leave 2 or 3 good follicles. The sperm injection or insemination is carried out immediately afterwards.

The advantages of IUI in contrast to natural conception, especially Medicated IUI, are that the timing of ovulation is monitored and enhanced; the IUI itself means that the sperm are delivered much closer to the 'target' eggs; often in medicated IUI cycles more than 1 egg is produced; and finally the sperm sample is washed and prepared prior to insemination.

Medicated IUI – need open tubes

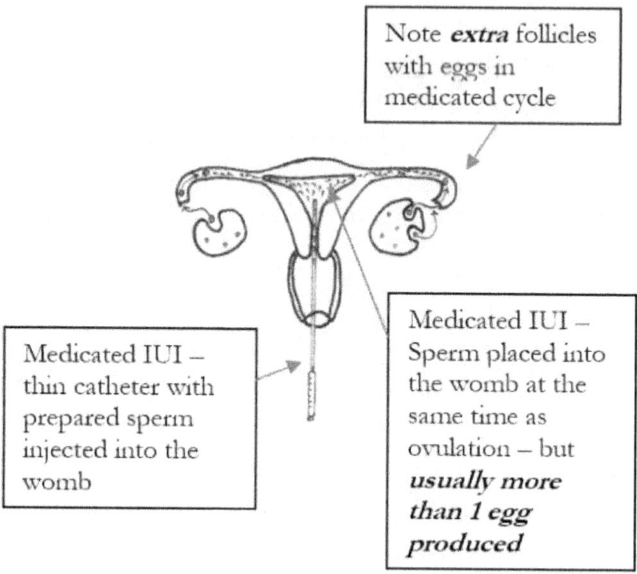

The insemination itself is a bit like having a smear. It should not be painful. A speculum is inserted into the vagina to see the cervix or neck of the womb. Then a soft flexible tube is inserted into the womb. The prepared sperm is then injected into the womb and hopefully the sperm and egg(s) meet and fertilisation takes place.

What are the success rates with IUI?

Success rates are difficult to judge because women have IUI for all sorts of different reasons. There is some evidence that IUI helps couples to conceive if the diagnosis is (i) Unexplained infertility, (ii) Endometriosis, (iii) Suboptimal sperm counts – although for IUI to be successful there must be at least 3-7 million viable motile sperm injected into the womb.

Success rates with Medicated IUI (partner):

Approx. Take Home Baby Rates – Medicated – **Partner IUI**	
<35 years old	13%
35-37 years old	13%
38-39 years old	10%
40-42 years old	7%
43 years old	Very low%

It is interesting that if **donor** sperm (as opposed to partner's sperm) is used, live birth rates with IUI do appear to improve certainly in women less than or equal to 37 years old. So particularly for same-sex couples using donor sperm in an IUI cycle, the table below is more representative:

Success rates with Medicated IUI (donor sperm):

Approx. Take Home Baby Rates – Medicated – **Donor IUI**	
<35 years old	18%
35-37 years old	15%
38-39 years old	11%
40-42 years old	5%
43 years old	Very low%

Before you have IUI, your doctor must ensure that your fallopian tubes are open and normal otherwise the procedure is a waste of time and money. This can be done with either an HSG test, a HyCoSy or a laparoscopy (See Chapter 4).

Finally, to qualify for IUI, the male partner must have at least

3-5 million motile sperm that be retrieved from the ejaculate; if it is less than this IVF/ICSI should be considered.

So, the message is:

1. IUI is a good initial treatment option for patients with Unexplained Infertility / Endometriosis / PCOS / Mild male factor subfertility / Same-sex female couples using donor sperm / Same-sex male couples using one of the partner's sperm with a surrogate.

2. It can be either a natural IUI cycle or medicated IUI cycle using *Clomid* / *Letrozole* or a Gonadotrophin (FSH).

3. It can be used to achieve pregnancy in same-sex female couples with donor sperm of their choice.

4. It can be used to achieve pregnancy in same-sex male couples using their own sperm and a surrogate.

5. The fallopian tubes must have been tested beforehand to ensure that they are open either by HSG or HyCoySy or Laparoscopy (keyhole).

6. IUI is cheaper that IVF (about one third of the cost) and so worth considering.

7. If you are not pregnant after 3 treatment cycles of IUI, it is time to consider possible IVF.

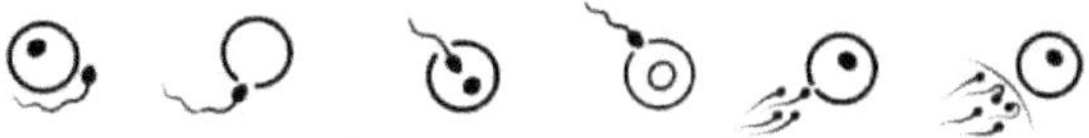

CHAPTER 5C

IVF (IN VITRO FERTILISATION)

What is IVF?

"In vitro" means "in glass". Fertilisation means the fusing of an egg and sperm to form an embryo. Hence, IVF is the fertilisation of the egg with sperm that occurs outside the body in a glass test tube. Hence the term "test tube babies".

"In its simplest terms IVF works like this — the woman is started on a daily injection that generally stops her own hormones working. Then an additional daily injection that stimulates her ovaries to grow lots of follicles (containing eggs) is started. After about 10-14 days of growth, these eggs are then removed from the ovaries via a needle through the vagina. The eggs are mixed with the male partner's sperm to form an embryo (test tube baby). The embryo(s) are then grown for a few days in the laboratory, in a specialised incubator under the care and watchful eyes of a team of embryologists. At the right time, one or more of the embryos are then drawn up into a small catheter and placed into the uterus or womb of the woman concerned. Hopefully the embryo then implants into the endometrial lining of the womb and two weeks later a pregnancy test is done."

So when is it appropriate to use IVF or ICSI?

Reasons for treatment with IVF

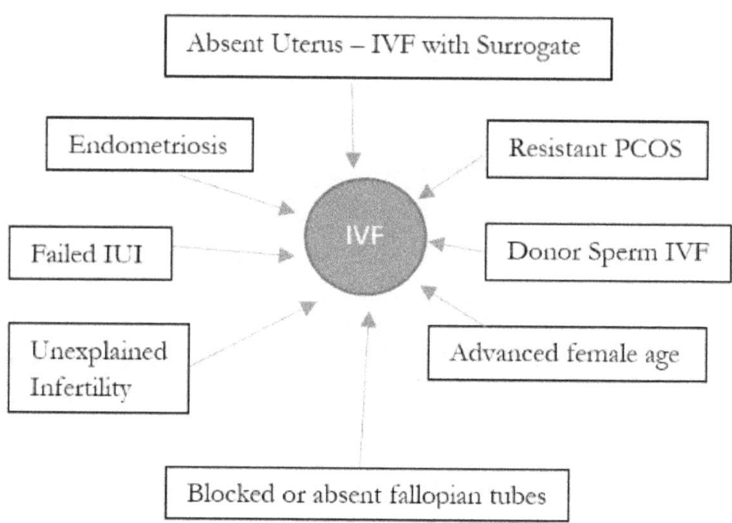

Damaged Tubes

Since IVF bypasses the fallopian tubes, any woman with damaged, blocked, or absent fallopian tubes can still get pregnant using IVF. For example – (i) women who have had previous PID (chlamydia) with blocked fallopian tubes, (ii) women who have had previous surgery to remove the tubes because of ectopic pregnancy, hydrosalpinges (dilated damaged tubes with fluid collection within) or endometriosis.

Failed IUI

If IUI treatment has failed after 3 cycles, most clinics would recommend the couple to have IVF which has better success rates.

Resistant PCOS

When the woman is not ovulating naturally, if she had failed ovulation induction and especially has undergone failed IUI.

Endometriosis

When there is inflammatory change in the pelvis and particularly if IUI has already failed, IVF is required. If the tubes are blocked or there are lots of adhesions (scar tissue around the ovaries) because of endometriosis, IVF is indicated.

Same-Sex Couples

Female: Many same-sex female couples opt for IVF with donor sperm. One of the partners elects to undergo IVF to produce the eggs. These are then mixed with donor sperm to form embryos, which can then be placed back into either of the partners' womb. Often, one of the partners produces the eggs, and the other acts as the recipient by having the created embryos placed back into her uterus. Any resulting pregnancy has enabled both female partners to have a hand in the "making" of their child.

Male: A male same-sex couple will need to find an egg donor and a surrogate uterus in order to achieve their dream of having a child. This can be done by fertilising donor eggs with one the male partners' sperm to form embryos, one or two of which are then transferred into the surrogate uterus.

Advanced Maternal Age

Since success rates are a great deal better when using IVF in comparison to IUI, many older women will elect to have IVF in preference. Certainly the older the eggs or the lower the AMH, the lower the chance of a successful pregnancy outcome. So, although it is more expensive, IVF will provide the best chance of pregnancy.

On occasions, if the woman has a very low AMH, or she is much older, IVF techniques can be used to produce embryos with DONOR eggs (from a younger woman) – these are then mixed with the partner's sperm to form embryos, one or two of which are placed back into the older woman's womb to achieve pregnancy. This often results in a positive pregnancy test since one of the biggest factors in achieving success, is the **age of the eggs**. If the eggs are from a young woman, the success rates should be good.

Reduced Sperm Counts

If the male partner has a markedly reduced sperm count, then although it is not impossible to conceive naturally or with IUI or IVF, the statistics are not good. Therefore ICSI (see Chapter 5D) is indicated.

Unexplained Infertility

A third of couples who cannot achieve natural pregnancy have completely normal investigations and there is no explanation as to why they cannot conceive. These couples will often start treatment with a few cycles of IUI, but if this does not result in a pregnancy will benefit from IVF. Some couples will elect to go straight for IVF and this is especially true if the couple have been trying to conceive for more than 2 years or the woman is 35 or more years old. IVF itself can sometimes diagnose why the couple cannot get pregnant – for example about 5% of unexplained infertile couples who have never achieved conception together have a problem when the egg and the sperm meet. None of the sperm, despite being present in their many thousands, are able to penetrate the egg. In this case although the process of IVF can yield eggs which are mixed with sperm, yet no embryos are formed. When this happens it is called "Failed

Fertilisation", since despite optimum conditions for eggs to be fertilised by the adjacent sperm, there appears to be an incompatibility. Such couples need a different form of IVF called ICSI (Intracytoplasmic Sperm injection – see Chapter 5D) when a single sperm is injected directly into the egg to achieve fertilisation.

In couples with unexplained infertility having an IVF cycle, we will often counsel a 50:50 IVF/ICSI split, such that if fertilisation via IVF fails, ICSI should work.

Absent Uterus

In some women, there might be a rare genetic condition where there is no development of the womb. Another scenario may be that a woman has had a hysterectomy for example because of a cervical cancer, but she stills retains her ovaries. In such cases, IVF can still be carried out and the resulting embryo/s can be transferred in to a surrogate womb.

Step-by-step guide to IVF (what physically happens)

There are a number of medication protocols or drug treatments used to stimulate the production of eggs but probably the most common treatment is known as the "Long Protocol" and it works like this:

(i)   After full assessment by medical staff and once the decision for IVF has been made, patients are invited to attend for "treatment planning". This will involve supplying medication (usually in the form of small injections – injected just under the skin, similar to injection of insulin in diabetic patients) and instructions on how and when to give the medication. Generally, the woman or her partner are taught to administer the medication. Dates for the start of your treatment that are mutually convenient are then decided and you are then ready to start.

(ii) Twenty-one days after the start of your period, you will be instructed to give yourself a small daily injection (a **GnRHa** – Gonadotrophin Release Hormone analogue – a common one is called *"Suprecur"*) that will be continued until the time of your egg collection. This medication is also available in the form of a nasal spray and some units use this in preference to the injection. A **GnRHa** is a posh name for a substance that is used to gain control over your natural cycle. It will stop you producing your own Follicle Stimulating Hormone (FSH) and Luteinising Hormone (LH) – this is called "Down Regulation" and means that the fertility clinic can control the growth and collection of eggs at the right time without interference from your own natural hormones. The **GnRHa** "downregulates" the production of your own fertility hormones.

(iii) Usually after 7-10 days of these (**GnRHa**) daily injections, you will have a period. At that stage you are invited back to the clinic for a "baseline" ultrasound scan. All scans carried out in fertility clinics use the transvaginal route. In other words, instead of the usual scan on your tummy, a slim probe is inserted into the vagina where excellent views of the endometrium, uterus, and ovaries are achieved. At the baseline scan it is important to check that the endometrial lining of the womb is reasonably thin (it should be because you have just had a period and the endometrium has been shed) and that there are no ovarian cysts present. Thereafter, you will be instructed to start the second daily injection **(Gonadotrophin – FSH or FSH+LH)** that will stimulate your ovaries to produce follicles (hopefully with eggs in them). Common Gonadotrophin preparations are called *"Menopur"*, *"Meriofert"*, *"Gonal F"*, *"Fostimon"*, *"Bemfola"* and *"Ovaleap"*. These are small daily injections given just under the skin, but usually in higher doses than you would produce naturally. So instead of just 1 follicle (with an egg in it) being produced as in a natural cycle, multiple follicles in both ovaries are stimulated.

(iv) The developing follicles are then monitored with regular ultrasound scans, watching them as they grow. When the maximum number of follicles have grown to around 18-22mm in diameter, they are ready for harvesting. At this point a single injection of LH or HCG is given in the knowledge that it will result in ovulation 36-40 hours later. Thereafter, a transvaginal egg collection is organised just prior to this in order to collect the eggs before ovulation.

Transvaginal Egg Collection

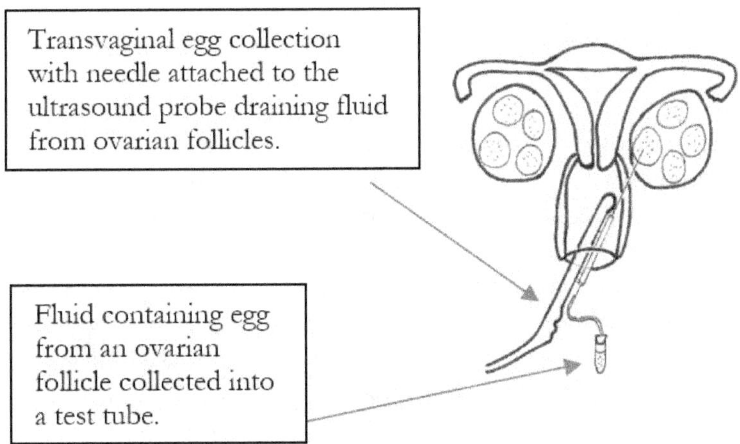

The egg collection is usually done under sedation using the equivalent of intravenous *Morphine* and *Valium*, so the patient is sleepy with good pain relief. Some clinics carry out the procedure under general anaesthesia. A slim ultrasound probe with a fine cylindrical bracket attached, is gently inserted into the vagina. A fine needle is then pushed through the bracket, and through the vagina under ultrasound guidance into each of the ovaries. Each follicle within the ovaries is then pierced with the fine needle and drained. Fluid from each follicle is collected into a test tube that is immediately examined for the presence of an egg, which is obviously retained. The whole procedure rarely last more than 20 minutes.

(v) Once collected, between one and four eggs are placed in a dish and exposed to between 100,000 and 200,000 sperm, one of which will then hopefully penetrate each egg and fertilise them to form the embryos. After their formation, the embryos are generally grown for a further 5 days in the laboratory to reach the "Blastocyst" stage. The embryologist will then choose one or two of the best embryos which are then placed back into the womb – the **Embryo Transfer**. The embryos will then hopefully implant into the endometrium and start to grow. Two weeks later a pregnancy test is carried out.

The **Embryo Transfer** (ET) procedure is usually very straightforward and the vast majority are done without sedation or anaesthesia. A speculum (the same as having a cervical smear) is inserted into the vagina, the cervix is located and washed before an embryo transfer catheter is inserted so that it lies 1cm to 1.5cm from the top of the endometrial cavity. This is usually done under ultrasound guidance. In this way the embryo(s) are subsequently gently injected into the endometrial cavity and thereafter the catheter is slowly and gently withdrawn. Often a 'dummy run' or practice Embryo Transfer is carried out either at the time of the egg collection or preferably in the month prior to the treatment cycle to ensure there are no potential problems with insertion of the ET catheter.

Embryo transfer

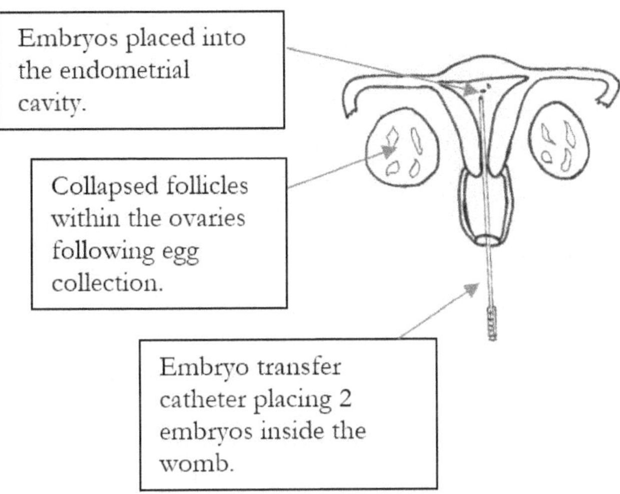

What happens if I have embryos left over? Frozen Embryo Transfer (FET)

Frequently patients have one or two embryos replaced into the womb, but have embryos left over from their IVF cycle. If these embryos are of good quality they can be frozen and then thawed at a later date for another embryo transfer (known as FET – Frozen Embryo Transfer). The successful thaw rate is approximately 95%. This means that if the fresh embryo transfer failed to yield a successful pregnancy or the couple just want another baby, they can have a FET without having to go through IVF all over again.

How many embryos can be placed into the womb?

The HFEA (Human Fertility and Embryology Association) encourage *single* embryo transfer to reduce the risk of twins and triplets. Put simply, having 1 embryo put back into the uterus significantly reduces your chance of having twins or triplets. With twins there is an increased risk of almost *everything.* For the mother – miscarriage/diabetes/pre-eclampsia, bleeding, and ultimately maternal death. For the baby – stillbirth, cerebral palsy, prematurity (in other words being born before 37 weeks). So having a single embryo put back into the womb to produce a single child seems sensible.

The HFEA states that no more than 2 embryos can be put back into the womb if the woman is under 40 years old at the time of the transfer. If she is 40 years old or more at the time of the transfer, then **up to** 3 embryos can be put back.

It is interesting to note that the **overall pregnancy rates are the same** whether 2 fresh embryos are put back into the womb or the woman has 1 fresh embryo transfer and if that does not work, a frozen embryo transfer at a later date. The overall cumulative pregnancy rates are the same but the significant risk of twins is avoided with the latter.

How do I know if my endometrial lining is receptive to the embryo(s) at Embryo Transfer (ET)?

A receptive endometrium (lining of the womb) is very important for implantation of the embryo(s) during the course of an IVF/ICSI cycle. As already described it is important to assess the endometrium with ultrasound before IVF to ensure there are no abnormalities such as polyps or fibroids indenting the endometrial cavity. Sometimes it is necessary to do a hysteroscopy (see Chapter 4). Thereafter, during the IVF cycle, there is some evidence that a thick and juicy endometrium appears to improve pregnancy rates. Some fertility specialists say that **the endometrium ideally should be at least 6mm to 8mm (on ultrasound) in thickness** to ensure a good chance of implantation, although pregnancies can occur even if the endometrial thickness is less than this. In addition, there is some evidence that if the **endometrial lining has a certain "Trilaminar" (3 layered) appearance**

at the time of the Hcg injection, pregnancy rates are better. Therefore, during your IVF cycle it is reasonable to ask your fertility doctor about the state of the endometrial lining as they see it on ultrasound.

Sometimes **the presence of free fluid within the endometrial cavity is thought to reduce the chance of a successful outcome** following embryo transfer. Free fluid can be visualised with ultrasound scanning prior to and at the time of the ET. If free fluid is present at the time of the ET, there are a number of options available: (i) Continue with the ET (ii) Use a fine catheter to try and withdraw the fluid from inside the cavity and then proceed with the ET (iii) Postpone the ET for another cycle by freezing the embryo(s) and doing an FET at a later date when hopefully the fluid is absent. This is a difficult decision, since putting in a catheter to withdraw fluid from the cavity can potentially damage the lining of the womb, and freezing the embryos is not always successful if they are not of a good quality. Thankfully this is relatively rare.

Finally, if you have had a number (usually 3 or more) of failed implantations, despite having good embryos – there is a relatively new test that looks at the receptivity of the endometrial lining to determine the best time for transfer. **This is called the ERA or Endometrial Receptivity Assay.** (Please see Chapter 9 for more information on ERA).

Do all the follicles seen on ultrasound scan contain eggs?

Not every follicle will contain an egg. Approximately 70% of follicles drained at egg collection will yield an egg. You cannot see an egg in the follicle on scan. The follicles must be drained and the follicular fluid collected is then viewed under the microscope by an embryologist to identify an egg.

What is a good number of eggs to be collected during an IVF cycle?

The optimal number of eggs to be collected is anything from 4 to 15 during an egg collection. Although what is really important is not the quantity of eggs retrieved but the quality. We have collected over 10 eggs in some women and they have failed to conceive, whereas others with just 2 or 3 eggs have gone on to have a healthy baby. As a general rule two thirds of eggs collected will fertilise and become embryos. So, if 10 eggs were collected, you would expect 6-7 of them to fertilise to form embryos. Once more than 15 eggs are collected, the risk of ovarian hyper-stimulation starts to go up (see Chapter 7 – Risks Associated with IVF).

How successful is IVF?

IVF success rates per cycle in the majority of women are approximately 20% to 35%. In comparison, a young fertile couple trying to conceive naturally have a 15% to 20% chance of conception per month of trying. IVF success rates vary depending on the age of the woman and her AMH. Also if she has had a baby in the past, success rates seem to improve.

Be careful to distinguish between "Take Home Baby Rates" and "Pregnancy Rates". Many women will get pregnant with IVF, but this does not equate to a baby in your arms because of the risk of miscarriage. The bottom line is not pregnancy rate, but "Take Home Baby Rate (THBR)". Below is a table giving approximate THBRs depending on age:

Approx. Take Home Baby Rates	
<35 years old	32%
35-37 years old	27%
38-39 years old	21%
40-42 years old	13%
43 years old	5%

From this very important table, you can see that if a couple go privately for IVF treatment, they will spend approximately £5,000 on a treatment that will, at best, realise their dreams of having a child about a third of the time. If the woman is 43 years old, the couple will spend significant amounts of their income on a procedure that is likely to fail 95% of the time! Although sometimes it appears harsh, it is important to be absolutely truthful with patients.

It is therefore massively important that the couple are aware of these statistics before investing physically, psychologically, and financially into Assisted Reproduction treatments.

What is IVF Lite?

IVF Lite is a milder form of IVF, which uses lower doses of drugs for shorter time periods and is co-ordinated within the natural menstrual cycle. The focus is on quality of eggs and embryos as opposed to the quantity of eggs and embryos. Some authorities believe that using lower doses of drugs may increase the quality of eggs and embryos, as well as achieving better implantation. In addition, the cost of the treatment is lower because IVF Lite involves less medication. Risks such as Ovarian Hyper-stimulation Syndrome (OHSS) are lower because the ovaries are not being overly stimulated.

In one particular American study, it was shown that minimal stimulation IVF gave similar results to conventional IVF but was much cheaper with fewer side effects. The same study suggested that in older women and those with very low ovarian reserve, IVF Lite was actually superior to conventional IVF, although for younger women it was slightly worse. The pregnancy rate per egg retrieved in all cases was higher with less stimulation, although of course fewer eggs are likely to be retrieved with IVF Lite.

So, the message is:

1. IVF success rates are dependent on many factors including age, AMH, and whether you have had a child before, but in a woman less than 35 years of age, the success rate is approximately 32% (national average) per cycle.

2. IVF is the indicated treatment if the tubes are blocked.

3. IVF is the next step if IUI has failed.

4. Consider going straight to IVF if you are older (> 35 years old or your AMH is low).

5. If you have enough eggs – you may have enough embryos for a fresh embryo transfer and still have embryos to freeze – this means you can have a FET (Frozen Embryo Transfer) later on without having to go through a whole cycle of IVF again.

6. Ask your fertility clinic doctor about your suitability for IVF Lite.

Even if using IVF – success rates drop dramatically with increasing female age – **DO NOT WAIT TOO LONG**.

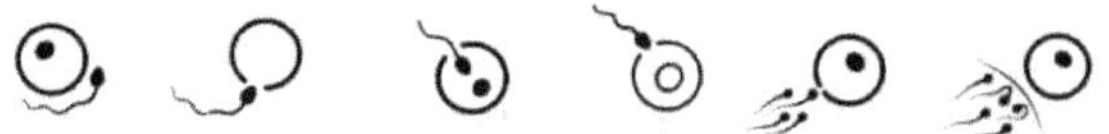

CHAPTER 5D

ICSI (INTRA-CYTOPLASMIC SPERM INJECTION)

What is ICSI?

ICSI or Intra-Cytoplasmic Sperm Injection is exactly the same as IVF except that following the egg collection instead of each egg being exposed to thousands of sperm, a single sperm is injected directly into each collected egg in the hope that fertilisation will take place and the embryo will form. The inside of the egg is called the *cytoplasm*, hence the term Intra-*Cytoplasmic* Sperm Injection.

Intra-Cytoplasmic Sperm Injection

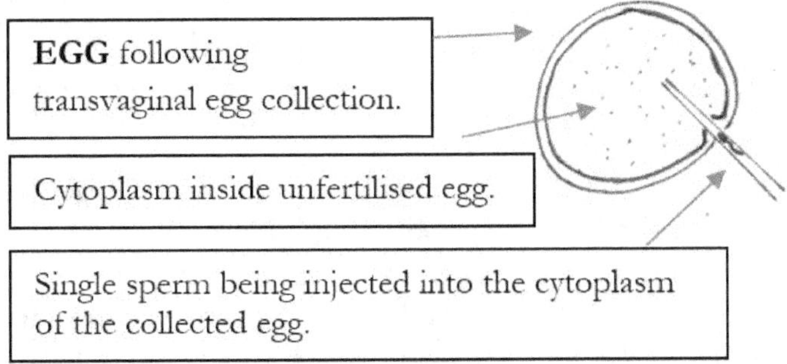

Hence, if the male partner has a markedly reduced sperm count, reduced number of moving sperm or poor quality sperm, it is still possible through the science of ICSI for embryos to be made and couples to fulfil their dream of having their own child. We can also perform ICSI with sperm that has been retrieved surgically where a patient has a blockage preventing sperm leaving the body or where sperm are in such low numbers that we can only obtain them surgically (please see Chapter 13).

As well as very poor sperm count, another reason for using the ICSI technique is when despite adequate numbers of sperm, fertilisation at IVF does not occur. About 5% of infertile couples who have never achieved conception together have a problem when the egg and the sperm meet. If eggs are placed with 100,000 to 200,000 motile sperm (which is the washed and prepared sample from the raw semen analysis) and no fertilisation takes place, it is understandably extremely upsetting for the couple involved. The only logical way forward at that point is to repeat the whole cycle but the next time to use ICSI instead of straight IVF.

The third use of ICSI is the fertilization of thawed frozen eggs. Some women will choose to have an IVF cycle to obtain eggs which they can then store for years until they are ready to have a family. Collection and storage of eggs maybe because of an illness (for example a cancer or chemotherapy) such that eggs are collected *before* any treatment which may harm the ovaries. Alternatively, a woman who is getting older and hasn't found the right partner may wish to store her eggs for the future.

When planning a treatment cycle, if there is any doubt about the sperm sample being good enough or there is the potential for failed fertilisation at IVF, then often couples are advised to go for a 50:50 split, whereby 50% of the eggs are fertilised with IVF, whilst the other 50% are fertilised with ICSI. This provides a reassuring backup in the case of potential failed fertilisation.

Following ICSI, the hope is that fertilisation takes place and embryos are formed. Thereafter, just as in the IVF procedure, one or two of the embryos are placed into the womb (embryo transfer). Implantation of the embryos into the endometrium then hopefully takes place and a pregnancy test is carried out 2 weeks later.

Reasons for treatment with ICSI vs IVF

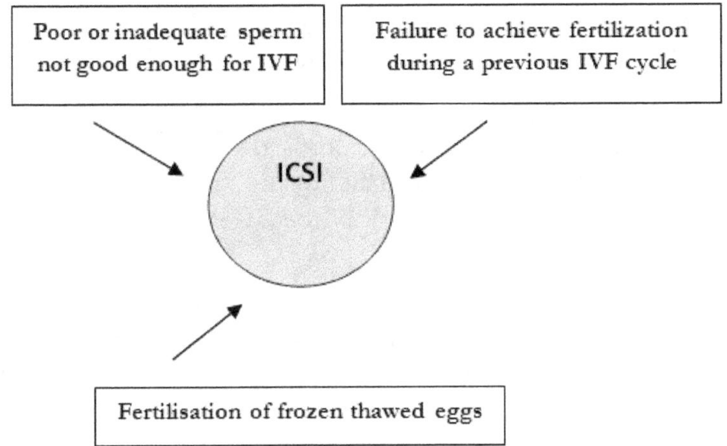

So, the message is:

1. ICSI is the same procedure as IVF, except that instead of thousands of sperm being placed with each collected egg, one sperm is directly injected into each egg to achieve fertilisation.

2. There are three main reasons to use ICSI instead of IVF and they are: (i) markedly reduced numbers of sperm and (ii) failed fertilisation in a previous IVF cycle and (iii) ICSI fertilisation of frozen thawed eggs.

3. When undergoing an IVF/ICSI cycle, some couples opt to have 50% of the eggs fertilised by IVF and 50% of eggs fertilised by ICSI. This means that if the IVF does not work (no fertilisation), the ICSI backup will still hopefully yield embryos.

4. Success rates are similar to IVF – but again the message is that success rates with ICSI drop dramatically with increasing female age – **DO NOT WAIT TOO LONG** before seeking help.

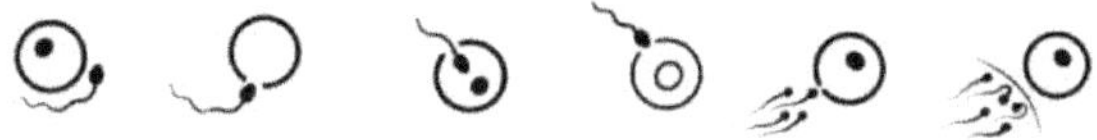

CHAPTER 6

ADVICE FOLLOWING YOUR EMBRYO TRANSFER

Couples often ask for advice following their embryo transfer, worried that certain activities may harm the implantation/growth of the embryos or that they may compromise the chances of success – here are a few basic dos and don'ts:

Can I pass urine after my embryo transfer (ET)?

The answer is categorically yes! Many women are afraid to have a pee after ET, because they understandably feel that they may wash the embryos out. Be reassured – this is impossible. The urine is stored in the bladder and exits through a small tube called the urethra. It is completely separate from the cervix and the womb, where the embryos have been placed. Pee to your heart's content, the embryo(s) are safe.

Can the embryo(s) fall out after ET?

When the ET is carried out the embryo(s) are usually placed 1cm to 1.5cm from the top of the womb, inside the womb cavity. But the womb cavity is not a voluminous space into which the embryo(s) are injected. It is a closed space, with endometrium lying on endometrium, analogous to a sandwich. The embryo(s) are then placed in between the layers of the endometrial "sandwich". It is most unlikely that they can fall out.

What should I eat/drink?

It is sensible to eat a healthy, balanced diet. Try to eat plenty of protein and avoid spicy foods and bowel irritants. Drink about 2 litres of fluid per day and avoid caffeine/alcohol. Ensure that you are taking Folic Acid (this needs to be started 3 months prior to conception) and continue this up to 12 weeks of pregnancy. Continue your medication as per the instructions of your IVF clinic.

Physical activity – what can I do?

Certainly for the first 3-4 days after ET, try and keep physical activity to a minimum, thereafter live life normally but avoid strenuous exercise and swimming certainly until the outcome of the treatment is known. Avoid sex until the outcome of the treatment is known.

Avoid stress

Although, to the best of our knowledge, there is no compelling evidence for this – it is sensible to avoid stressful situations in either in work or at home.

What happens if I have a bleed after the Embryo Transfer?

Light vaginal bleeding can occur following implantation of the embryo, so not all vaginal bleeding is bad news – women can sometimes bleed quite heavily and still be pregnant, so the best advice is to carry on with the above and your medication until the pregnancy test on day 14-16 following the ET. If you bleed very heavily, however, or have what feels like a normal period – the pregnancy test is likely to be negative.

Once the pregnancy test is positive and then I have a bleed, how do I know if I have miscarried?

Bleeding in early pregnancy is quite common and does not necessarily mean the end of the pregnancy. Once you get to 5-6 weeks gestation, contact your clinic or GP who can organise an ultrasound scan. We have scanned many women who have had bleeding in early pregnancy and the scan findings still showed a normal pregnancy inside the uterus. Even after vaginal bleeding, if a foetal heart is seen on ultrasound – approximately 90% of those pregnancies continue.

However, if a woman experiences pain as well as bleeding in early pregnancy it is likely that she is miscarrying. If this occurs seek MEDICAL HELP, especially to rule out an ectopic pregnancy (pregnancy implanted into the tube) which can be life threatening.

What medication is used after ET?

Commonly, progesterone is used following ET. These medications act by stabilising the lining of the womb and there are a number of different types:

(i)   Utrogestan 200mcg pessaries – these are usually placed in the vagina, x3 per day until 12 weeks of pregnancy.

(ii)   Cyclogest 400mcg pessaries – these are usually placed in the vagina x2 per day until 12 weeks of pregnancy.

(iii)   Gestone Injection (50mg/100mg) – this is a daily injection until 12 weeks of pregnancy. It is an intramuscular injection (deep into the muscle) and it is our experience that women find it more painful to administer than preparations that are subcutaneous (injected just under the skin).

(iv) Lubion Injection (25mg) – this is a daily injection until 12 weeks of pregnancy. It is a subcutaneous injection (injected just under the skin) and it is our experience that it is less painful to inject than intramuscular injections.

(v) Crinone Vaginal Gel – this is a vaginal gel which is inserted into the vagina with an applicator once or twice per day up to 12 weeks of pregnancy.

Some patients **may** also be given other medication which are individually tailored depending on the patients' history and circumstances. They include:

(i) *Clexane* (40mg) injections daily if history of recurrent miscarriage (3 consecutive miscarriages) and investigations show an abnormality of the woman's blood tests.

(ii) *Prednisolone* (5-20mg tablets daily) if history of recurrent miscarriage.

(iii) *Oestradiol* (2mg tablets) – if there is a history of poor thickness of the lining of the womb.

(iv) *Aspirin (75mg or 150mg)* – especially if history of recurrent miscarriage with Antiphospholipid Syndrome.

So the message is:

1. Congratulations – you have got to this stage having undergone an IVF/ICSI cycle and embryo(s) have been successfully created by the joining of egg(s) and sperm. The embryo(s) have now been put back into the best incubator in the world (your womb). Now it's that long two-week wait before the pregnancy test. But so far so good.

2. Post transfer, it is all about being sensible:

   Eat well
   Sleep well
   Rest
   Avoid stress

3. Take your medication as prescribed.

You have done your best and hopefully will now be rewarded.

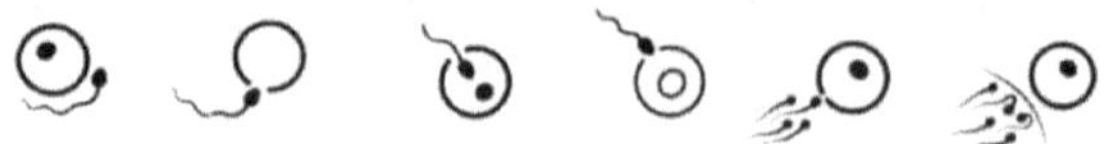

CHAPTER 7

RISKS ASSOCIATED WITH IVF/ICSI

We wrote this chapter, because from time to time we see couples who merrily waltz into clinic with an unrealistic idea that modern medicine and fertility techniques can sort out any problem and cure any ill – this is just **not** true. Expectations can be massively high and disappointment completely unexpected. Whilst it is true that millions of IVF babies have been born since the birth of the first IVF baby (Louise Brown) in 1978, it is also true that IVF can be a difficult path to tread where more often there is more disappointment than joy. If you are contemplating infertility treatment do so from a realistic and well informed perspective.

Psychological, Physical and Financial Trauma

Infertility Treatment… "If successful there are very real and joyful rewards. Even if unsuccessful, IVF often draws a line in the sand, after which a couple can reflect, 'we can sleep easy knowing that we tried everything to have our own child'." But there are very real psychological, physical, and financial implications and risks.

The whole process of going through a fertility treatment has very real implications for the psychological and physical well-being of the couple involved. From the initial investigations all the way through to the long wait for the positive pregnancy test. The journey may involve surgery, for example to remove a polyp from the lining of the womb or indeed an ovarian cyst, and this is before the IVF treatment has even started. The use of medication to stimulate the ovaries is not without its risks in terms of not only general discomfort but also more serious scenarios such as Ovarian Hyper-stimulation Syndrome (OHSS). The transvaginal egg collection carries risks of bleeding and infection, as well the discomfort of a needle into the pelvis and ovaries. The drugs used to either sedate or anaesthetise during the egg collection can induce nausea and vomiting. On occasions the embryo transfer itself can be traumatic, particularly if there is difficulty negotiating the cervix to place the embryo(s) into the correct place within the womb.

The psychological stress on the couple undergoing IVF can be enormous. The drugs themselves can make the woman emotionally vulnerable. Ultimately the necessary exposure of your most personal, intimate self – both psychologically and physically – can be hugely unsettling. The waiting for results of investigations, the understandable fear of various procedures such as egg collection, and then the wait and hope for a positive pregnancy can all be hugely stressful. The cruelty of a positive pregnancy test followed by a miscarriage is a massive kick in the teeth when the couple are already on an emotional rollercoaster. The whole process can put a strain on personal relationships, induce feelings of depression, and inevitably on many occasions tears are shed.

There are important financial implications too. In the UK, the average cost of an IUI treatment is £1,000 per cycle. The cost of an IVF treatment cycle can be anything from £3,500 to £6,000. If ICSI is required, a further £700 to £1,200 can be added to the cost. Following an IVF treatment cycle, if there are embryos suitable for freezing, then a future FET (Frozen Embryo Transfer) will cost approximately £795 to £1,300. So it is important to point out that as well as the physical and psychological trauma, there will be a financial hit as well. Our experience of this is that you need to be savvy.

Know what your limits are and stick to them. Be careful about possible hidden extra costs, for example like cost of drugs/embryo storage/extra embryology techniques like assisted hatching. Ensure that hidden costs are exposed so that total expenditure can be assessed and budgeted for. Finally, if you are lucky enough to live in the UK, remember that you are entitled to free NHS fertility treatment (although this is postcode dependent), although that entitlement may change if you have had private treatment. It is also important to know same-sex female couples may well be entitled to NHS Donor sperm-IUI or Donor sperm-IVF, although it would appear that same-sex male couples are not entitled to the NHS treatment with a surrogate, which does seem unfair. Often the couples concerned are not aware of the various NHS entitlements and more worryingly, their GPs are sometimes not aware either.

The Risk of Failure of Treatment

At the risk of sounding like a merchant of doom and gloom, it is important to point out that on average, even in the best hands IVF will yield a "take home baby rate" of about 33%. That means approximately two thirds of the time, an IVF cycle will not work. It is also important to point out that when a clinic publishes its pregnancy rates, this may not equate to the all-important "take home baby rate". This is because of the risk of miscarriage. This, on average, affects between 15-20% of all pregnant women and goes up significantly with age.

Ovarian Hyper-stimulation Syndrome (OHSS)

What is OHSS and how often does it occur?

OHSS is a real problem with infertility treatment and a potential nasty side effect particularly in young women with

Polycystic Ovarian Syndrome. It is essentially overstimulated ovaries from the gonadotrophins (FSH) used to stimulate the growth of follicles in the ovaries. The overall approximate risk of getting OHSS is about 4%. The severest form requiring admission to hospital happens in about 0.5% to 1%.

What are the symptoms of OHSS?

In OHSS, the ovaries become enlarged and the blood vessels in the body become leaky. This results in fluid leaking out of the blood vessels into the abdomen and sometimes lungs. The abdomen can then become swollen and tense, leading to discomfort and sometimes pain. Hence women experience bloating, nausea, and vomiting. Occasionally fluid leaks out into the lungs to cause breathlessness. In addition, women with OHSS are more likely to get blood clots in their legs, arms, neck, or even head, resulting in pain in the affected area or even headache.

How many types of OHSS are there and how long will it last?

There is early or late OHSS. Early OHSS occurs shortly after egg collection (3-7 days). Late OHSS happens following a pregnancy test (12-17 days) and is usually more severe and associated with pregnancy (which causes ongoing stimulation of the ovaries by producing HCG). The OHSS can last from a few days to a few weeks.

Can OHSS cause death?

The short answer is yes, but it is very rare – approximately 1 in every 425,000 IVF cycles.

How is OHSS treated?

Following IVF/ICSI or even stimulated IUI cycles, if you get any symptoms of bloating, abdominal pain, nausea or vomiting seek help from the clinic where you had your treatment. The HFEA (Human Fertilisation and Embryology Authority) stipulate that patients having IVF should have 24-hour-a-day access to help. Most cases of OHSS are very mild and resolve with ensuring that adequate fluid is drunk (at least 2 litres of fluid per day) and high protein diet/drinks. Sometimes painkillers/anti-sickness medication is required. Many patients are given a "blood thinner" injection (*Clexane*) which prevents the formation of blood clots. If OHSS is severe, admission to hospital with intravenous fluids, blood tests, and strict monitoring is required. Occasionally, the fluid in the abdomen builds up too much it will need to be drained by a thin tube inserted into the abdomen.

If a woman is high risk for OHSS, how can it be avoided?

The risk of OHSS can be reduced by using low doses of gonadotrophins (FSH), particularly in younger women or those with a previous history of OHSS. If during the cycle there are multitudes of follicles (certainly more than 15-20) with free fluid seen in the abdomen on ultrasound, the cycle can be abandoned. Alternatively the cycle can continue and egg collection can be carried out but all the embryos are frozen. By avoiding a fresh embryo transfer, the patient cannot get late OHSS (usually the more severe form) and then the embryos can be safely frozen and replaced at a later date (as a FET – Frozen Embryo Transfer) when everything has settled down.

Will OHSS affect future cycles?

If you have experienced previous OHSS, then the drug

regime used in any subsequent cycle will need to be carefully chosen and the patient monitored even more closely during that cycle. Sometimes the patients are pre-warned that frozen embryo transfer may be more likely in any subsequent IVF cycle.

Risk of Egg Collection

During collection, a needle is inserted through the vagina into the pelvis which forms part of the abdominal cavity. As well as the ovaries and uterus, loops of bowel are present and the operator must take care not to needle the bowel. In addition, there are a number of large blood vessels adjacent to the ovary and any needle must stay well clear of these structures.

Risks are therefore those of potential bleeding and infection. Very rarely, following an egg collection a laparotomy (operation involving surgical opening of the abdomen) is required to fix any potential problems caused by egg collection. Many fertility clinics will give antibiotics prior to egg collection to prevent infection.

There are occasions where the ovaries are so high that they cannot be safely accessed using the transvaginal route. This is why the baseline scan is so important to ensure that the ovaries are accessible.

Multiple Pregnancy

In the UK, the transfer of more than 2 embryos in women under the age of 40 is not allowed. Guidance from relevant UK authorities encourages single embryo transfer where at all possible. The reason for this is that multiple pregnancies carry significantly increased risks in comparison to singleton pregnancies.

What are the risks in an early twin pregnancy?

Increased risk of late onset OHSS.

Around 30% of twin pregnancies reduce to singleton pregnancy – in other words one of the babies die.

What are the risks later on in a twin pregnancy?

The perinatal mortality (death rate) and morbidity (disease or disability) rates in twins are approximately 5 times that of singleton pregnancies. Preterm delivery (earlier than 37 weeks) is 3 times more common with twins than with singletons and a major problem with preterm delivery is Respiratory Distress Syndrome (breathing difficulties).

The risk of stillbirth in twins is approximately twice that of singleton pregnancies. There is a fourfold risk of cerebral palsy in twins with increased risks of brain haemorrhage and asphyxia. There is a greater risk of congenital abnormalities in twins.

For the mother the risks go up as well. There are increased risks of anaemia, high blood pressure, pre-eclampsia (otherwise known as Toxaemia), abnormal bleeding during the pregnancy, postpartum haemorrhage, and birth complications. Because of the much greater risks to mother and babies, twin pregnancies are always under the care of a consultant obstetrician in the UK and the pregnancies need much greater monitoring with regular scans and antenatal follow-up.

The psychological consequences for families then having to come to terms with handicapped children and the effect that it has on the immediate and wider family should also be taken into account.

What about triplets and beyond?

Hopefully you have got the picture with regard to the increased risks of twins. With triplets and beyond, the risks go up even more. In fact in some countries, "Foetal Reduction" or the removal of one or more of the foetuses at 9-12 weeks of pregnancy is carried out to reduce the risks. This can cause miscarriage in up to 15-25% of cases.

How can I reduce my risk of multiple pregnancy?

This is easy – have a single embryo put back. It is also true to say that if the remaining embryo(s) are good enough to freeze and the woman comes back at a later date for a frozen embryo transfer – THE OVERALL PREGNANCY RATES ARE THE SAME.

Are children born by IVF/ICSI more likely to have congenital birth defects?

Worldwide, millions of babies have been born by IVF, and the vast majority of these babies are fine. However, a number of studies suggest that fertility treatments like IVF and ICSI **do** increase the risk of congenital abnormality in comparison to babies conceived naturally. Abnormalities of the heart, genitals, anus, and nervous system (spina bifida) are all included in this, and it is interesting that congenital abnormalities appear to be more frequent after ICSI than IVF.

However, it is very important to put this increased risk into context. The background congenital abnormality rate in naturally conceived babies is approximately 5%, and following IVF/ICSI, it is increased by approximately 1 to 2% (thus to a congenital abnormality rate of approximately 6% to 7%).

All pregnant women in the UK are offered an anomaly scan to look for structural problems of the heart, bowel, kidneys, limbs, spine, etc. This is usually timed for 18-20 weeks into the pregnancy. It is significant that **no additional** screening for congenital abnormalities in babies conceived by IVF/ICSI is carried out, because the increased risk is perceived to be too small.

Are children born by IVF/ICSI more likely to have genetic abnormalities?

There is an increase in unrecognised genetic abnormalities in those needing IVF/ICSI treatments. For example, in men with very low numbers of sperm, chromosomal abnormalities can be anything up to ~13%. Microdeletions (absence) of parts of the Y chromosome (part of the DNA that determines sex) can be present in up to 15%. When ICSI is used because of abnormal sperm (patients with very low sperm counts – male factor), there does appear to be an increase in abnormalities of the sex chromosomes of children born and sub-fertile men with specific chromosomal abnormalities may pass on the same fertility problems to their sons. Some men with very low unexplained sperm counts may also be **carriers of the cystic fibrosis** gene. This means that although they themselves do not have the cystic fibrosis disease, they may pass on the defective gene to **any offspring**. If their partner also has the defective gene, then any resulting children may inherit the actual cystic fibrosis disease. Hence, it may be sensible for men **who have very low, unexplained sperm counts to consider genetic testing.**

Women who require IVF/ICSI may also be more likely to have genetic abnormalities, but there is rarely any screening unless there is a strong personal or family history.

What can I physically do to reduce the risk of congenital abnormality?

There is evidence that smoking cigarettes, drinking alcohol, and using recreational drugs in pregnancy can increase the risk of congenital abnormalities – SO DON'T.

The first 12 weeks of a pregnancy is probably the most important time to avoid medication and drugs. This is because it is during this time that the internal organs of the developing baby are being formed. After 12 weeks most of the major structures are already formed and now only have to grow. If possible it is always advisable to consider a reduction or stopping some types of medication during the first 12 weeks of pregnancy, *but only after consultation with your doctor.*

Plenty of rest is important. Healthy diet and light exercise is good. Avoid vitamin supplements not designed for pregnancy – for example vitamin A in excessive amounts has been found to cause congenital defects.

Finally, we always ask patients to ensure that they are on Folic Acid. There is evidence that this significantly reduces the risk of conditions like spina bifida in unborn babies. It needs to be taken before conception to make sure that it is in the system, as well as during early pregnancy.

So, the message is:

1. Infertility treatment is not without its risks. It is costly, physically and psychologically draining.

2. Be realistic – approximately two thirds of the time, each IVF cycle will not work and the success rate declines with age.

3. Since twin or triplet pregnancies are much higher risk than singleton pregnancies, carefully consider having a SINGLE embryo transfer to reduce this risk.

4. Be aware that there is an increased risk of congenital abnormalities in babies born by IVF/ICSI, but the vast majority of babies born are still normal.

5. The use of various medications for Assisted Reproduction do have side effects and the various procedures including transvaginal egg collection are not without risks.

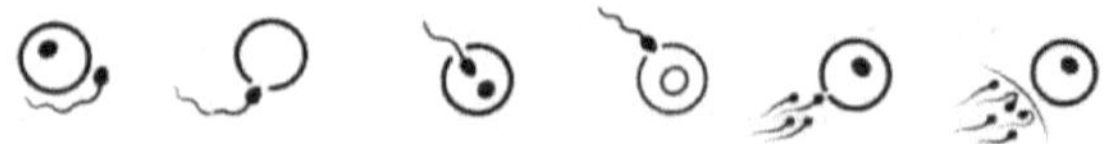

CHAPTER 8

EARLY PREGNANCY AND ANTENATAL CARE FOR PATIENTS HAVING IVF/ICSI

Once couples have achieved their dream of becoming pregnant through assisted reproduction treatments, they then have hopefully 9 months of pregnancy before the big day of their baby's birth. This chapter is designed to inform and advise on some of the potential problems that may need to be overcome during your pregnancy.

Early Pregnancy Problems –

1. The single biggest risk in early pregnancy is that of miscarriage which occurs 15-20% of the time. Women can present with bleeding or pain or both and clearly it is a very frightening and traumatic time, and help both physical and psychological should be available. We have seen many patients with a threatened miscarriage who present with painless bleeding, and on many occasions when they have been scanned the baby's heart is actively beating and all is well. In such patients, it is important to point out that despite the early bleeding, **if a scan shows a live pregnancy the outcome is usually very good with approximately 90% of pregnancies reaching a successful outcome.** So, in the event of some painless bleeding do not automatically assume that all is lost. Pelvic pain and bleeding together are a great deal more worrying. Miscarriage and recurrent miscarriage will be covered in some detail in Chapter 10.

2. Another risk in early pregnancy is that of an Ectopic Pregnancy which is when the embryo implants outside the uterus, usually in the fallopian tube (approximately 95% of the ectopic pregnancies are tubal, although some embryos implant in an ovary or elsewhere). Ectopics occur in approximately 1.4% of all pregnancies. They occur more commonly in patients who have had a previous ectopic, or pelvic infection, or previous tubal surgery. With IVF pregnancies there is an increased risk of something called a **Heterotopic Pregnancy** which is when one embryo implants in the uterus, but another one outside the uterus (usually in the tube) – so one normal pregnancy and one ectopic. Clearly this is more likely if more than one embryo was transferred in an IVF cycle and your doctor needs to be aware of this possibility.

3. Ovarian Hyper-stimulation Syndrome (OHSS). This has already been discussed in Chapter 7, and is unique to patients having stimulated cycles in Assisted Reproduction. What is important for you and your doctor to be aware of is the fact that patients who have suffered with **severe OHSS** may be more likely to experience high blood pressure during pregnancy and may be more likely to go into premature labour. Monitoring and awareness of this is therefore important.

4. Hyperemesis (nausea and vomiting in early pregnancy). This is very common in pregnancy with 80-90% of all women experiencing some nausea and vomiting. Reassuringly, for most it gets better after 12-16 weeks gestation. However, about 2% of pregnant women will experience severe nausea and vomiting where they cannot keep any fluid or food down. As such they become dehydrated and unwell, with symptoms of light-headedness, dizziness, exhaustion, thirst. This is called

Hyperemesis Gravidarum. It is treated with anti-sickness medication, vitamins (B6 especially), sometimes steroids and if the woman is unable to keep any fluid down, she will need hospital admission and intravenous fluids (a drip) to rehydrate her. If a pregnant woman becomes dehydrated she will be at a higher risk of thrombosis (blood clots) and this needs to be prevented with special medication. Unfortunately, once you have had hyperemesis, you are more likely to get it again in any subsequent pregnancy. **A little bit of nausea and vomiting in pregnancy is very common, but if you are unwell and not able to keep any fluid down – seek medical advice.**

After assisted reproduction treatments, many Fertility Units will offer and organise an ultrasound scan at approximately 6-7 weeks gestation in the event of a positive pregnancy test. Thereafter, patients with early pregnancy problems are usually **looked after in an NHS facility, commonly known as EPAUs (Early Pregnancy Assessment Units)** who will see, assess, scan and give advice and ongoing treatment to women with symptoms, in particular that of pain and bleeding. This is usually from 6 weeks onwards. Therefore, if you have a problem, see your GP who will usually arrange for you to be seen in an EPAU.

Much of the screening for problems like Down's syndrome in early pregnancy are based around the gestational age of the growing foetus. **As such, it is important to remember that the gestational age of the baby is taken from the date of the egg collection, not the embryo transfer.** This is important because as well as ensuring accurate dates for screening in early pregnancy, it allows for an accurate estimated date of delivery.

Later Complications

It should be pointed out that approximately 1-5% of all babies born in developed countries are as a result of IVF/ICSI (Assisted Reproduction) and in the majority of these, there is a normal outcome, so be reassured. However, there does appear to be an increase in the risk of some complications and you and your doctor should be aware of these. It is thought that some of these complications occur more frequently because women undergoing IVF/ICSI may be older, with higher BMIs, may have Polycystic Ovarian Syndrome (PCOS) and are more likely to present with multiple pregnancies in the form of twins or even triplets.

Pregnancies resulting from IVF/ICSI may have a greater risk of:

1. **Pregnancy Induced Hypertension** (PIH – basically high blood pressure in pregnancy) and Pre-eclampsia (otherwise known as Toxaemia – dangerous condition where the blood pressure goes up, but also protein is found in the urine) – **ALL patients should be screened for risk factors for this and if they are high risk should be offered daily Aspirin (75-150mg daily) from 12 weeks gestation.** Thereafter, regular screening in your antenatal checkups throughout the pregnancy should be carried out, monitoring your blood pressure and checking your urine for protein.

2. **Gestational Diabetes** (diabetes during pregnancy) – this is important to test in women who have a history of **Polycystic Ovarian Syndrome (PCOS) who have twice the risk of developing diabetes in pregnancy** – it is usually tested with a blood test that measures the amount of sugar in your blood when you have fasted and after a sugar load – it is called a "Oral Glucose Tolerance Test (OGTT)".

3. **Blood clots (or thrombosis)** – this often presents with a pain or swelling in your lower leg or calf muscle, the risk of blood clots goes up anyway in pregnancy irrespective of whether you have had IVF/ICSI. But certainly if you get symptoms of pain/redness/swelling in the calf or you are short of breath (sometimes blood clots can go to the lungs and cause shortness of breath) seek medical attention. Your doctor/midwife should look at various risk factors including your age (high risk if older than 35 years old), BMI (higher risk if >30 kg/m^2), smoking habits, presence of varicose veins, family history of blood clots, twins (or multiple pregnancy) or any innate tendency to form blood clots. **If you are high risk you will be offered blood thinning agents to prevent blood clots forming. Be aware of this and ensure you are checked out.**

4. **Growth restriction of the unborn baby** – this means that the baby's growth is compromised and is potentially associated with the baby not doing so well. There is some evidence that IVF/ICSI is associated with slowing down of the growth of babies when they are in the womb, although in the UK, it is considered to be a **minor risk factor** and no additional surveillance in the form of growth scans with ultrasound is recommended solely on this basis. However, other **minor risk factors** should also be taken into account:

a. Maternal age more than 35 years old
b. Nulliparity (i.e. first baby)
c. BMI between 25 and 29.9 and BMI < 20 (i.e. thin)
d. Smoker (1-10 cigarettes per day)
e. Previous history of Toxaemia (pre-eclampsia)

Some of the above are going to be quite common in patients undergoing fertility treatment, and the advice is that **any woman with 3 of these minor risks** (so for example IVF pregnancy/first baby/BMI = 27) would need an extra scan at 20-24 weeks gestation and this would need to be repeated in the third trimester (in the latter stages of the pregnancy).

Listed below are major risk factors for growth restriction and **if any woman has one major risk factor, she will need serial regular growth scans (scans approximately every 3 weeks) throughout the pregnancy.** You will note that one of the major risk factors is maternal age of 40 years old, which again is relatively common in patients undergoing IVF / ICSI.

Major risk factors for growth restriction during your pregnancy:

a. Age 40 years or more
b. BMI>30
c. Smoker >11 cigarettes per day.
d. Drug user (cocaine)
e. Diabetic
f. High blood pressure
g. Other medical problems, for example kidney disease
h. Heavy bleeding during your pregnancy
i. Abnormalities of some other blood tests
j. History of being a small baby in the mother or father

All the above constitute a high risk for the baby's growth slowing down and as such serial growth scans should be organised.

1. **Increased risk of Stillbirth.** This is the big one – there is some evidence that pregnancies conceived via IVF/ICSI have a **doubling of the stillbirth rate** which obviously is a potential disaster. As such, many

obstetricians would recommend that pregnancies are induced at term (from 37-40 weeks gestation), to get the baby out. Other obstetricians will be happy to continue the pregnancies with ongoing regular surveillance and monitoring. The risk of stillbirth in any case goes up with increasing gestation – so that stillbirth is more common at 41 weeks then it is at 39 weeks. Also stillbirth is increased with increasing maternal age. It is **important to discuss this thoroughly with the obstetrician looking after you to sort out a plan for when you will be delivered and how.** Remember you are **absolutely entitled to have an elective caesarean section** after frank discussion of the relative risks. Some women are not aware of the fact that they have this choice.

2.   Other risks include an increase in the risk of **preterm labour** (i.e. the baby decides to come out early) and potential problems with the placenta or afterbirth and these should be appropriately monitored during the course of your pregnancy.

It is so important to state that most pregnancies conceived by IVF/ICSI proceed normally, but the aim of this chapter is to make you aware of some of the possible complications and you can therefore discuss matters with your health providers with some knowledge. Importantly try and avoid multiple pregnancy (Twins and Triplets) by considering single embryo transfer or at least having a thorough discussion with your doctor at the time of your IVF cycle.

The authors' opinion – should pregnant women who have had infertility treatment be regarded as high-risk patients?

It is our opinion that the answer to this is categorically yes. In patients who have had IVF, or even just a past medical history of infertility, there is an increase in the risk of smaller growth-retarded babies, early delivery (prematurity), and stillbirth in comparison to women who have conceived spontaneously.

The authors' opinion – should pregnant women conceived by IVF be under consultant-led care?

Again, in view of the above, the answer is yes. Additionally, it is our opinion and practice to ensure growth scans are carried out in such women to ensure that the unborn baby's growth and wellbeing are monitored. The risk of stillbirth goes up with increasing gestation – so that stillbirth is more common at 41 weeks than it is at 39 weeks. Also, stillbirth is increased with increasing maternal age. Hence, it is our opinion that as a general rule, delivery of these patients should be timed for between 39 and 40 weeks – but not later.

So, the message is:

1. Early pregnancy problems following IVF include miscarriage, ectopic, OHSS, and hyperemesis. After discharge from your fertility unit, these problems are dealt with in specific Early Pregnancy Assessment Units (EPAUs) in your local NHS hospital and your GP.

2. Multiple pregnancy (Twins and Triplets) should be avoided by having a Single Embryo Transfer – the risks of virtually all complications goes up significantly with multiple pregnancy.

3. Pregnancies resulting from IVF/ICSI may have an increase in the risk of High Blood Pressure/Pre-Eclampsia/Blood Clots/Growth Restriction of the baby/Stillbirth – although some of this may be related to the age and medical history of the woman. In any case ensure you are aware of the risks and are adequately screened and monitored.

4. There is some evidence that the risk of Stillbirth goes up in pregnancies conceived by IVF/ICSI. The risk of Stillbirth is higher at 41 weeks gestation than it is at 39 weeks gestation in any case. Be sure to discuss timing of delivery with your health professional.

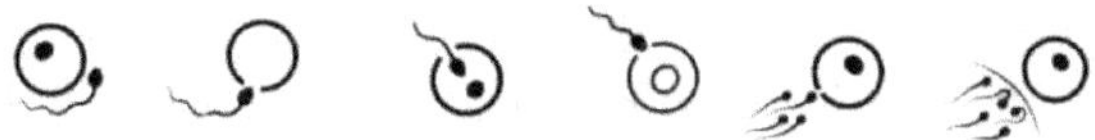

CHAPTER 9

WHAT ELSE CAN I DO TO IMPROVE MY CHANCES OF GETTING PREGNANT AND HAVING A SUCCESSFUL IVF OUTCOME?

On the internet and in the fertility literature there are all sorts of suggestions to improve your chances of conception, and we wanted to simplify these with a few words on each and advice on whether you should utilise them.

Please note that the HFEA (Human Fertilisation and Embryology Authority) have devised a "Traffic Light Rating" system for treatment add-ons, such that 'Green' is where there is *good* evidence, 'Amber' is where there is *conflicting* evidence and 'Red' is where there is no good evidence to show that any add-on treatment is effective in **most** fertility patients with regard to improving the chances of having a baby. The HFEA website is provided at the end of this chapter. Be aware that some of the add-on treatments are relatively expensive and may have side effects.

Endometrial scratch

This really is what it says on the tin – a scratch of the lining of the womb. The woman has a speculum placed into the vagina (just like when you have a smear) and a thin straw-like tube (called a *Pipelle)* is inserted through the cervix into the womb. The end of the *Pipelle* has a small sharp opening which essentially "scratches" the endometrium, traumatising it in the process. The procedure is carried out in the second half of the cycle (day 19-26) prior to the forthcoming treatment cycle. It is always sensible to take some painkillers (e.g. *Paracetamol* or *Ibuprofen*) about 1 hour beforehand. The procedure is done in clinic, takes about 5 minutes, and you go home about 20 minutes afterwards. Because the lining of the womb is being scratched sometimes you can experience some bleeding vaginally – this is not uncommon and nothing to worry about. In order to have this procedure you need to make sure that you are definitely not pregnant for obvious reasons.

So why do it? It is thought that one of the factors that prevents pregnancy is failure of the embryo to implant into the lining of the womb – this may be because of a poor quality endometrial lining. If a couple produce good quality embryos and then IVF consistently fails to make the woman pregnant it seems logical to assume that the problem may be with the endometrial lining. There have been some studies in the scientific literature to show that endometrial scratch can improve the implantation rate in women with repeated IVF failures. However, recent studies showed no difference in outcomes with endometrial scratch – therefore careful discussion with your fertility doctor is needed. The HFEA have traffic lighted endometrial scratch as AMBER.

Endometrial Receptor Assay (ERA)

For patients who have experienced recurrent implantation failure following embryo transfer, there is a relatively new personalised test that looks at how receptive the lining of the womb or endometrium is for implantation of the transferred embryo(s). The test involves taking a biopsy (just like an endometrial scratch) of the endometrium during a woman's natural cycle or during a medicated cycle and analysing it genetically, to determine if it is "receptive" or "non-receptive" for implantation of an embryo – this then provides guidance as to when to replace a frozen embryo or donor embryo during the time period of "receptivity" in a subsequent cycle. This technology may help to optimise the timing of embryo transfer, particularly in women who have had recurrent implantation failures. However, the HFEA has traffic lighted ERA as RED at the current time and careful discussion with your fertility doctor is needed.

Intra-lipids

This is basically a bag of liquid fat that is given intravenously (a drip in the arm) around the time of your IVF treatment and post embryo transfer. The theory is that this treatment reduces the NK (Natural Killer) cell population which some people say might affect implantation and miscarriage. There has been little evidence to show that intra-lipids improve pregnancy and live birth rates in women having IVF who have had recurrent implantation failure/miscarriage and who have increased NK cells. It is given "off label" (in other words, not like a normal prescription) and the HFEA has traffic lighted the use of Intra-lipids as RED at the current time and careful discussion with your fertility doctor is needed. In addition, there can be significant side effects with its use.

DHEA (Dehydroepiandrosterone)

DHEA (Dehydroepiandrosterone) exists as a natural hormone in the body that is relatively abundant at around the age of 21, and then significantly drops in concentration with increasing age. DHEA is one of the building blocks or precursors to a number of important hormones needed for reproduction. Since DHEA drops with age and is related to hormone production, researchers have wondered if fertility is improved by taking DHEA supplements, particularly in older women.

One study found that by taking three 25mg tablets of micronized DHEA for 3 months before starting IVF stimulation, there was a significant increase in the pregnancy rate. The results suggested an improved ovarian function in poor responders and those over 40 years old by taking DHEA. There is also evidence that DHEA reduces chromosomal abnormalities if taken as a supplement one to three months prior to IVF, which in turn may reduce the risk of miscarriage.

So DHEA taken as the micronized form 75mg daily for 3 months prior to IVF treatment may:

(i)   Increase IVF success rate
(ii)   Increase egg/embryo numbers
(iii)   Decrease spontaneous miscarriage rates
(iv)   Reduce chromosomal abnormalities

However, taking this medication may result in oily hair and skin. It is also important to remember that there is still controversy regarding treatment with DHEA, with some authorities still not convinced of its effectiveness and regarding it as experimental. It is always worth seeking advice from your fertility clinic/doctor before taking this supplement.

What are the authors' views on DHEA?

After looking at the evidence for the use of DHEA, although not absolute, there does seem to be some evidence for its use. However, we would not use it as a first line and we would not use it if there had been an adequate response to the IVF drugs in a previous cycle. We would, however, think about using DHEA for 3 months prior to an IVF cycle IF there had been a previous poor response in previous cycles.

Where can I get DHEA from?

Internet suppliers of micronized DHEA

Co-Enzyme Q10

Co-Enzyme Q10 or Ubiquinone is a substance that naturally occurs within the body, which appears to diminish in concentration the older we get. Its function is to help generate energy within the cells of the body. The human egg is a large cell that when penetrated by a sperm has lots of little "factories" (the biological name for these factories is Mitochondria) that produce lots of energy to drive the development of a normal embryo. One *theory* is that the older the egg, the less Co-Enzyme Q10 these little factories contain, and so the less energy the fertilised egg can produce to drive the development of a normal healthy embryo. Supplementation of the diet with Co-Enzyme Q10 may *theoretically* enhance the performance of these little factories within the egg to improve energy production and hence provide a positive effect on the genetic material within the fertilised egg to improve egg quality and implantation.

Co-Enzyme Q10 is not a prescription medication, and can be bought over the counter. It is being used by a number of older women undergoing IVF to theoretically improve their egg quality. More scientific research needs to be done to determine if it is really helpful in improving egg quality – but there is no evidence to date that it does any harm if taken before an IVF cycle in doses of 200mg daily.

Impryl

Impryl is a nutritional supplement used in both men and women with fertility issues. **There is evidence that the micronutrients within Impryl improve live birth rates in couples with a history of infertility,** by potentially improving egg and sperm quality. This nutritional supplement is certainly worth considering and is available to buy through the internet or from fertility units that stock it. The authors of this book would recommend the use of Impryl.

Testosterone/Testosterone Patches

There is some evidence that the use of testosterone gel applied to the skin (transdermal) can increase the live birth rate in IVF patients who were previously found to be poor responders if used 3-4 weeks before the start of IVF cycle. Again, we would not use testosterone *unless* there had been a poor response in previous IVF cycles. Discussion with your IVF doctor is warranted about its use in the event that you do not respond to the medication to stimulate your ovaries.

Steroids

Steroids are widely used in medicine to treat inflammatory conditions – so for example, if you have eczema – steroid cream (Hydrocortisone) is used; if you have asthma – steroid inhalers are used. In some patients the production of antibodies against their own body parts can cause an inflammatory response that can affect their fertility. For example, some women may produce antibodies against their own ovaries (anti-ovarian antibodies) or against their thyroid gland (anti-thyroid antibodies). There is some evidence that the use of steroids in such cases when women have previously had recurrent implantation failures **may be** beneficial. In addition, although there may be side effects, it is unlikely that low-dose steroid tablets (for example Prednisolone 5-10mg) will do any significant harm, if given over a relatively short time period.

What are the authors' views on steroids?

In the event of a patient having previous failed cycles, in addition to an inflammatory condition with circulating antibodies against her ovaries or thyroid gland or others – we would certainly consider the use of a small dose (5-10mg) of steroid during a subsequent cycle after careful discussion with the patient concerned. However, the HFEA have traffic lighted the use of steroids as RED at the current time. Again, careful discussion with fertility doctor is needed.

Aspirin

Aspirin seems to be the "cure all" for a great many conditions. For example there is evidence that it acts to reduce the risk of bowel cancer, reduce the risk of strokes, reduce the risk of a repeat heart attack, and reduce the risk of thrombosis (formation of blood clots). It acts by reducing inflammation as well as being a "blood thinner". Some authorities feel that because it acts as a blood thinner it may improve the blood supply to the ovaries and improve ovarian response in IVF treatment. There is, however, NO good evidence that Aspirin can improve your chances when undergoing IVF. In fact there is some evidence that Aspirin can actually reduce your chances of ovulation, implantation, and increase your risk of bleeding.

However, if you suffer from **Recurrent Miscarriage Syndrome** (defined as three miscarriages in a row) AND you suffer from a condition called Antiphospholipid Syndrome (see Chapter 10 on miscarriage), then once pregnant, there is some evidence that Aspirin can help improve your chance of successful outcome of a live birth.

If given, Aspirin is usually given as a low-dose tablet of 75mg daily. It is available over the counter and does not need a prescription. However, you should seek advice from your clinic or doctor before using it. There are side effects including allergic reactions, upset stomach, heartburn and an increase risk of bleeding – although if used in a low dose (75mg), side effects are usually minimal.

What are the authors' views on Aspirin?

Generally, we would not use Aspirin in women undergoing an IVF cycle. The HFEA has traffic lighted the use of aspirin as

RED in an IVF cycle. Furthermore, we would not use Aspirin in early pregnancy since there is some evidence that it can increase the risk of miscarriage in the early stages, **UNLESS** there was a diagnosis of Recurrent Miscarriage Syndrome (3 consecutive miscarriages) and/or a diagnosis of Antiphospholipid Syndrome.

It is interesting that there is some relatively good evidence that in susceptible individuals, Aspirin reduces the risk of preeclampsia (or toxaemia) in pregnancy and certainly patients who are high risk for this (especially if they are already suffering from high blood pressure) should be given Aspirin in pregnancy – usually from 12 weeks gestation).

Clexane (Low molecular weight Heparin)

Clexane is a substance that essentially "thins" the blood and makes it less "sticky". It is a small injection usually given on a daily basis. In mainstream medicine, it is used to prevent and to treat thrombosis (formation of blood clots). It is safe to use in pregnancy. There is some evidence that in women who have a tendency to develop blood clots (the scientific name for this is thrombophilia), and in women with Recurrent Miscarriage Syndrome (with a condition called Antiphospholipid Syndrome), *Clexane* can be beneficial in improving live birth rates if given from the day of embryo transfer until birth. The usual dose is *Clexane* 40mg injected daily.

It is also interesting that *Clexane* has a role in modifying the immune system and preliminary studies have suggested that it might be useful when used with steroids in patients undergoing IVF, particularly if there is a history of "inflammatory conditions".

What are the authors' views on *Clexane?*

In patients with a history of recurrent miscarriage or a tendency to form blood clots (thrombophilia), the use of

Clexane makes absolute sense and we have a LOW threshold for the use of prophylactic low-dose *Clexane* following IVF and throughout pregnancy. Side effects include irritation at the site of injection, thinning of the bones (osteoporosis) after prolonged use, hair loss (very rarely), and reduction of platelets (a component of the blood that helps with formation of blood clots). This last side effect is very rare and we have never seen it in patients that we have treated. Periodic blood tests to check the platelets is sensible. Some doctors recommend the use of calcium tablets (500mg twice per day) to help prevent bone thinning if *Clexane* is taken for prolonged periods of time.

Embryological Factors (Please also see Chapter 14)

The Embryoscope

This is a cutting-edge embryo incubator that essentially employs time-lapse photography to film the progress of the developing embryos. A photograph is taken on a regular basis so that development of each embryo from the time of fertilisation to the time of embryo transfer is recorded. Hence, when each embryo is ready to be placed back into the womb not only can the embryo be graded according to what it looks like now, but also the development of each embryo from the earliest stages can be assessed. If there has been abnormal development noted by reviewing images from the Embryoscope, then that embryo is less likely to produce a viable pregnancy. On the other hand, if the embryo has shown normal development as witnessed by the Embryoscope, then it is more likely to yield a viable pregnancy. In this way the Embryoscope provides more information on how to choose the best embryos for embryo transfer to improve the chance of a positive pregnancy test and ongoing pregnancy. The HFEA has traffic lighted the use of time lapse photography as AMBER. Certainly there is no evidence of any harm.

Assisted Hatching

Around each embryo is a shell just like the chick in a bird's egg. Just as the chick needs to hatch out of its shell, so too does the human embryo need to hatch out of its own shell in order to implant into the lining of the womb. It is thought that one of the reasons that there is failure of implantation of the embryo is because that embryo has failed to hatch out of its shell. This is easily remedied by a procedure called "Assisted Hatching". This is carried out by a qualified embryologist who essentially holds the embryo and with the use of fine laser makes a tiny hole within the shell of the embryo prior to embryo transfer, which facilitates hatching. In the right hands, there is very little risk to the embryo, although the risk of identical twins is increased by a tiny amount (about 1%). Assisted Hatching is usually recommended if the female partner is more than 40 years of age, if the embryologist thinks the egg shell looks particularly thick, and finally if there is a history of failed implantation in previous cycles. The HFEA has traffic lighted the use of embryo hatching as RED because there is no evidence that it improves pregnancy rates for most patients. However, some clinics believe it is useful for certain subgroups of fertility patients. Again discussion with your fertility doctor is advised.

Embryo Glue

This is a great marketing name, but is certainly nothing like glue. The embryos can be placed into "Embryo Glue" prior to their transfer into the womb. Embryo Glue contains a substance called "Hyaluronan" which may improve the chances of implantation. Some embryologists feel that there is a small advantage to using this prior to embryo transfer. The HFEA has traffic lighted the use of Embryo Glue as AMBER and certainly there is no evidence of any harm.

PGT-A or PGS

PGT-A stands for Pre-implantation Genetic Testing for Aneuploidy. Aneuploidy means abnormal number of chromosomes for example, as seen in a person with Down's syndrome (who has an extra Chromosome 21). PGT-A used to be called PGS, which stands for Pre-implantation Genetic Screening. Anyhow, this is a process that occurs in IVF or ICSI cycles after the egg collection and formation of any embryo(s). From each embryo a cell or cells are taken and examined for genetic (chromosomal) abnormalities. Thereafter, only the good embryo(s) – or those without genetic (chromosomal) abnormalities are replaced back into the uterus. The procedure is intended to improve pregnancy success rates and reduce miscarriage rates, however to date, there is little evidence to show that PGS improves success rates in older women (who are more likely statistically to have a miscarriage) or those with recurrent miscarriage. Furthermore, the HFEA has RED traffic lighted this potential "add-on" to an IVF cycle. In other words, they say that there is no evidence from studies that it improves your chance of having a baby for *most* fertility patients. It is also relatively expensive. However, there may be some patients in whom it could be considered and thorough discussion with your fertility consultant is required

IMSI

IMSI stands for **Intracytoplasmic Morphologically selected Sperm Injection**. In English, this means that when the embryologist is looking for the best single sperm to use for injection, they use a special microscope that is x6000 more powerful to assess each sperm. In this way tiny defects in the sperm that would not ordinarily have been seen are detected and only "perfect" sperm used to inject into the egg. However, there is lack of good evidence to suggest the benefit of IMSI although some observational studies showed an improved pregnancy rate and a reduction in miscarriage rates. Recent Cochrane review (which roughly translated means 'a respected scientific evaluation of the situation') does not *support* or *refute* the clinical use of IMSI. The HFEA has RED lighted IMSI as an "add on" because there are doubts about its effectiveness. That having been said, there may be some patients in whom it could be considered and thorough discussion with your fertility consultant is required.

What are the authors' views on these Embryological Factors?

We would look carefully at individual patient circumstances to individualise the potential use of these procedures where indicated.

Acupuncture

The use of acupuncture in improving IVF outcomes is debatable and unproven. Generally, there is no good scientific evidence for its use that we can find in the scientific literature. However, we are aware that anecdotally, a number of women find it useful and certainly there is no evidence that it does any harm.

Pre-existing Medical Complaints

It is important any pre-existing medical or surgical condition is reviewed before embarking on a pregnancy. This is important for a number of reasons. The first is that poor control of certain medical conditions can have a very real adverse effect on the proposed pregnancy. Poorly controlled diabetes can increase congenital abnormalities and miscarriage. There is an association with abnormal thyroid function and miscarriage/infertility. Epilepsy and in particular the drugs used to treat it can have an adverse effect on the pregnancy. Drugs used to treat depression can have an effect on the development of a baby's heart. Drugs used for all sorts of other medical conditions can have an adverse effect on not only your chances of a successful IVF cycle, but also your chances of a successful ongoing trouble-free pregnancy. So the message is, seek medical help to effectively treat whatever condition that you have, and ensure that the medication used to treat it is pregnancy friendly.

Lifestyle Factors to help you get pregnant

Obesity – carrying excess weight correlates with menstrual cycle disturbance and infertility. Weight loss of just 5% can result in restoration of ovulation in some women with deranged menstrual cycles. The advantages of maintaining a healthy weight are obvious. There is evidence suggesting that **raised BMI can be associated with adverse outcomes with fertility treatments in terms of lowered success rates and increased miscarriage rates.**

Alcohol – excess alcohol can lead to disorders of ovulation and even stop a woman having periods altogether. Alcohol consumed in early pregnancy can lead to physical malformations, mental retardation, and growth restriction. There is some evidence that if you stop drinking alcohol completely you improve your fertility. In IVF cycles, consumption of alcohol was associated with reduction in pregnancy rates and increased miscarriage rates. It is also interesting that consumption of alcohol in the male partner was also associated with a reduction in achieving an ongoing pregnancy.

Smoking – there is evidence that smoking reduces ovarian reserve (kills off eggs), reduces the chances of getting pregnant, and reduces the chances of a fertility treatment being successful. Moreover, smoking during pregnancy increases the risk of miscarriage, increases the risk of preterm labour, increases the risk of growth restriction of the baby – this is easy – DO NOT SMOKE.

Diet – a good diet is important and eating well not only supports you, but also your baby during any subsequent pregnancy. Avoid processed foods that usually have extra salt and sugar. Eat unprocessed foods with plenty of fresh fruit and vegetables, meat, fish, eggs, pulses, nuts and other foods like pasta, rice and potatoes. If possible choose low-fat and low-sugar options (like semi-skimmed milk instead of full-fat milk). Choose unsaturated fats and oils and eat them in small amounts. Also **a recent new study has found that a Mediterranean diet may significantly boost women's (especially non-obese and <35 years of age) chances of becoming pregnant through IVF.**

As an aside remember there are some foods **best avoided once you are Pregnant:**

(i) Uncooked sausages, burgers, especially pork, since they may contain *Toxoplasmosis* bacteria – which is harmful to the pregnancy.

(ii) Liver and liver-containing foods that contain high amounts of Vitamin A, which again can be unsafe in pregnancy.

(iii) All types of pâté – they may contain *Listeria*, a bacteria that can be harmful to pregnancy.

(iv) Any food that is undercooked, unwashed or unpasteurised.

(v) Soft cheeses with white coating such as Brie or Camembert, as well as soft blue cheeses such as Danish blue – again there is a small chance they contain *Listeria*.

Statistics

It is important to remember that statistics play a major role in successful IVF/ICSI outcome. In the best hands and optimum conditions (young age, good AMH, no medical or surgical problems), pregnancy rates of 50-60% are seen, with "take home baby" rates of about 30-40% per cycle. This means that more couples are disappointed following an IVF cycle than are elated. Find out what the expectations for your age group are and be realistic about your chances. Sometimes the best thing you can do is be persistent and have another cycle. However, this needs to be put into context – we would not advise this in a 43-year-old woman who has an approximate 5% chance of a successful outcome in any IVF cycle using her own eggs. **A lot of the time, the answer is in the age of the woman and more precisely her eggs.** Hence the paragraph below on the use of donor eggs.

Use of Donor Eggs

Probably the single most important factor in determining the success of any IVF procedure is a determinant that the couple can do nothing about – **age, or more specifically the age of the eggs.** As already stated, many women leave it too late to start their family. After 35 years of age, a woman's fertility significantly reduces and her miscarriage rate significantly increases. IVF appears to be more successful at achieving pregnancy per cycle than natural means, yet at the age of 43, a woman has approximately a 5% chance of having a baby with IVF. That means she is going through a procedure that is costing her emotionally, physically, and financially with a 95% chance that it will not work. Furthermore, if she is more than 45 years of age, she has an approximate 93% chance of miscarriage. So, what is to be done to help that couple achieve the dream of having their own child? The answer is to use donor eggs. Utilising the eggs of a young woman fertilised by your partner's sperm is much more likely to give rise to a successful outcome. There are a number of factors we often quote to couples when they are deciding on whether to use donor eggs.

How similar is the genetic material between my eggs and those of a would-be donor?

The answer is that 99.5% of the genetic material between 2 human beings is the same. So when a couple state that donor eggs are not the same as their own they are right, but only 0.5% right – the rest of the genetic material is the same.

Can the embryo derived from a donor egg and growing in me be affected by the environment of my womb?

The answer to this question is absolutely yes. The growing embryo is influenced by your hormones, your blood supply to the uterus, your nutrition, and the environment in which the embryo grows. The pregnant woman shapes and determines the baby's future which carries 99.5% of her genetic material in any case.

Is the baby conceived by a donor egg really the recipient's baby?

The embryo already has 99.5% of his or her mother's genetic material. The embryo grows within that mother's womb, under the influence of her hormones, nutrition, blood supply, feelings, thoughts, and dare we say it, love. The mother then goes through labour and gives birth to deliver her baby. Is this her baby? We think so.

So, the message is:

1. If you have a pre-existing medical or surgical condition, it needs to be optimised. For example, if you are diabetic, good control before pregnancy can have a massive effect on reduction of miscarriage and congenital abnormality. Likewise pre-pregnancy review of other medical conditions is a must.

2. Alter lifestyle factors. Avoid smoking, drinking alcohol, and aim for a normal body weight.

3. Be aware of the success rates of IVF according to your age and AMH, if you are an older woman consider the use of donor eggs. Remember that donor eggs carry 99.5% of your own genetic material.

4. If you have a history of recurrent miscarriage or have an inflammatory condition, consider the use of a small dose *Clexane*/steroids.

5. If you are older, and have a history of poor response to medication given to stimulate your ovaries, consider using DHEA/Testosterone gel.

6. Remember IVF is a statistics game, ask your chance of success and plan accordingly.

7. If there was any one magical factor that made a huge difference to IVF success rates – everyone would use it. That having been said *it is* worth considering some off licence* options that may help to promote success rates.

*In the UK, prescribed medicines have a license to be used for particular conditions or illnesses. If a medication is used "Off-licence" it means it is being prescribed in an unusual and unlicensed way. Some medications utilised in the hope that they will improve IVF outcome (DHEA, Steroids, Testosterone, *Clexane*) are often used anecdotally and off-license. It is advisable to check with your GP or Fertility Doctor before using them.

Further information on fertility treatment "Add-Ons" can be obtained from the HFEA (Human Fertilisation and Embryology Authority) at:

https://www.hfea.gov.uk/treatments/treatment-add-ons.

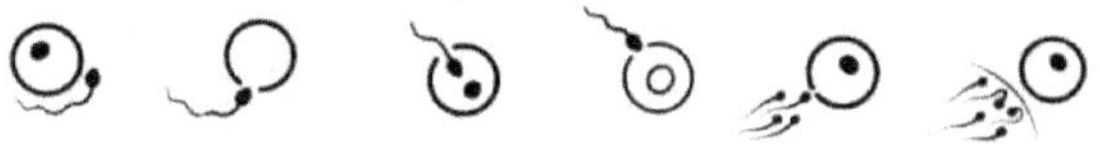

CHAPTER 10

MISCARRIAGE

How common is miscarriage?

Overall 15-20% of pregnancies end in miscarriage. That means up to every 5th woman you see on the street has miscarried.

Miscarriage is a cruel and heart-breaking phenomenon, but is massively common in the general population. The older the woman becomes, the more common it is. You will remember that unlike men who make new batches of sperm every 3 months, a woman is born with a finite number of eggs and these age as the woman gets older, so that by the time the woman gets into her 40s her miscarriage rate goes up considerably.

Again, the message is:

"If at all possible have your children before you reach 40 years of age."

The next table illustrates this point, such that if you are in your early twenties, your miscarriage rate is approximately 11%, whereas once you reach 40 years of age it is approximately 50%. These figures speak for themselves.

Age Range	Miscarriage Rate
Up to 19 years old	13%
20-24 years old	11%
25-29 years old	12%
30-34 years old	15%
35-39 years old	25%
40-44 years old	51%
>45 years old	93%

Table 8.1 Approximate Miscarriage Rate according to Maternal Age

When we see couples who have been through a miscarriage, many women will feel that they have done something wrong, eaten or even thought something they shouldn't have, and that they are responsible for the loss of their baby. They **unfairly blame** themselves for this frequent phenomenon and sensitive, supportive care is hugely important, together with an acknowledgement of the trauma of their loss.

So what does cause the majority of miscarriages?

The majority of miscarriages (up to 60%) are because of DNA or chromosomal abnormalities in the developing foetus or baby. The older you are, the greater the risk. For example, a woman's age-related risk of having a baby with Down's syndrome is approximately 1 in 1,000 when she is 30 years old, but it is 1 in 100 when she is 40 years old – a tenfold increase. Some couples will take a small amount of solace from the fact that although miscarriage is a very distressing time, sometimes miscarriage may be kinder than the eventual birth of a deformed or genetically abnormal baby.

It is also true that the age of the father contributes to the possibility of miscarriage, although is much less significant. It is thought that once the man's age goes beyond 40 years old, the risk of miscarriage starts to go up.

General lifestyle advice for optimisation against the risk of miscarriage

There is evidence that some fundamental lifestyle habits are associated with miscarriage. These include cigarette smoking, consumption of alcohol, and the consumption of coffee may also increase the rate of miscarriage. Avoidance of these precipitants, together with a good healthy diet, avoidance of rigorous exercise would clearly be sensible (and we do not mean going out for a jog a few times a week, we mean vigorous exercise – like running 20 miles three times a week!). In addition, there is evidence that being overweight (BMI>35) increases the risk of miscarriage and therefore lifestyle changes to address this are warranted.

If I have miscarried once already, what is my risk of miscarrying in my next pregnancy?

It is important to know, however, that if a woman (less than 35 years of age) has 1 miscarriage, her risk of miscarrying in the next, second pregnancy is still of the order of 15-20%.

If I have miscarried twice in a row, what is my risk of miscarriage in my next pregnancy?

If the same woman miscarries the second pregnancy, then her chance of miscarriage for the third pregnancy still remains about the same (15-20%).

If I have miscarried three times in a row, what is my risk of miscarriage in my next pregnancy?

When a woman has miscarried 3 times in a row she has a diagnosis of ***Recurrent Miscarriage Syndrome*** **(RMS)**, and now the chance of a future pregnancy miscarrying is of the order of 40%. Hence, RMS is defined as 3 miscarriages consecutively and is a syndrome present in 1% of the female population. This needs to be medically investigated.

It is important to state that the 40% risk of miscarriage is only present if there have been 3 consecutive miscarriages. If for example you have had 2 miscarriages followed by a normal pregnancy with delivery of a healthy child, and thereafter suffer from another miscarriage – this is not recurrent miscarriage syndrome. It has to be 3 consecutive miscarriages one after the after.

What are the other causes of miscarriage?

As already discussed, the majority of miscarriages (up to 60%) are because of DNA or chromosomal abnormalities in the developing foetus or baby, and the older you are the greater the risk. This does not mean that the pregnant woman or her partner have abnormal chromosomes, it is merely when the egg and sperm get together there is a mismatch of genetic material and the chance of this happening increases with the increasing age of the egg. To confirm that this has occurred you can ask for the products of conception passed during miscarriage to be sent off for genetic analysis.

When a miscarriage occurs three times in a row then as already stated the diagnosis is that of Recurrent Miscarriage Syndrome and investigations need to be carried out. There is no reason why your GP cannot do this for you. Hence the causes of RMS are as follows:

(i)   **Antiphospholipid Syndrome** – this is a posh name for a condition that occurs in approximately 15% of women with RMS and is important because it is **treatable.** A blood test specifically looking for this can be done by your doctor. Left untreated the chance of a live birth is only about 10%. With treatment, it is estimated that the chance of a successful pregnancy outcome is 80%.

(ii) **Genetic/chromosomal rearrangements of the parents** – this occurs in approximately 4% of couples with recurrent miscarriage. If the genetic testing of the products of conception show a particular sort of chromosomal abnormality then testing of the parents is carried out. This, again, is a blood test. If this test is positive for a genetic re-arrangement then the next step is to see a genetic counsellor who can advise on the best way forward.

(iii) **Congenital abnormalities of the womb** – some women have a split or partitioned womb (septate uterus), others may have a double womb (Uterus didelphys), or even half a womb (Unicornuate uterus) – these may increase the risk of miscarriage and preterm labour. This is usually identified with an ultrasound scan. Some women will require a hysteroscopy to further review this or even a MRI scan before deciding the best way forward. Any woman with a congenital abnormality of the uterus will need to be looked after in a consultant-led obstetric team during any pregnancy.

(iv) **Weakness of the cervix (or neck of the womb)** – this is often referred to as 'Cervical Incompetence' and usually manifests itself because the miscarriage occurs in the second trimester (between week 12 and week 24 of the pregnancy) after the neck of the womb in essence opens up with loss of the baby. Regular scans of the cervix to ensure that it remains closed are important and if it starts to open as seen on ultrasound, a timely stitch can be inserted into the cervix to keep it closed.

One important reason for weakness of the cervix can be a previous treatment following an abnormal smear. Every woman in the UK is invited to have a 5-yearly **smear and if this is abnormal, then they are invited to attend a special clinic called a Colposcopy Clinic. In Colposcopy, the doctor or nurse views the cervix by looking down a colposcope (essentially a pair of binoculars) that magnifies the cervix and helps them to see any abnormality – in particular pre-cancerous change. Often a biopsy is taken and if this shows pre-cancerous change (something called CIN – Cervical Intra-epithelial Neoplasia) then a treatment to remove that area is carried out. This is called a "Loop Excision" or LETZ (Large Excision of Transformation Zone) or sometimes a "knife cone biopsy". These treatments, particularly if carried out on more than one occasion, may significantly shorten the cervix and hence may make miscarriage and preterm labour more likely. In the event of pregnancy be sure to inform your obstetrician of any such treatments in the past – they may want you to have regular scans during your pregnancy (usually from 12-14 weeks onwards) on the cervix to ensure the cervix remains closed – if it does not then a cervical stitch can be put in.

(v) **Hormone factors** – this can be divided into 3 main categories:

a. The first is diabetes. Uncontrolled diabetes with high sugar levels is associated with miscarriage and foetal abnormalities. However, once identified and treated, the trend for miscarriage and foetal abnormalities is reversed. A simple blood test (HbA1c) carried out on the mother can look for this.

b. The second is thyroid disease. An overactive thyroid gland gives rise to symptoms of diarrhoea and weight loss. An underactive thyroid gland gives rise to symptoms of being cold, tired, and constipated. Both under and overactive thyroid disease can result in miscarriage. A simple blood test (TFTs – Thyroid Function Tests) can be carried out. Treatment of thyroid disease can reduce the risk of miscarriage.

c.   Polycystic Ovarian Syndrome. This can lead to a "diabetic-like" state which is thought by some to increase the risk of miscarriage. Therefore the antidiabetic medication Metformin has been used to treat women with PCOS who have had recurrent miscarriage, although the evidence that this helps is limited. However, there is no evidence that Metformin does any harm in pregnancy.

(vi)   **Immune Factors** – There is much talk of "Natural Killer" (NK) cells that exist in the bloodstream and in the uterus (endometrial lining) that may affect pregnancy and abnormalities of these may cause miscarriage. This is very much research based at present. Abnormal NK cells in the bloodstream are not thought to have any effect on miscarriage, however there is a link between abnormal NK cells in the endometrial lining of the womb and miscarriage. The use of steroids (for example *Prednisolone*) has been shown to reduce the numbers of abnormal NK cells in the endometrial lining but has not been associated with any reduction in miscarriage rates. Despite this, some doctors recommend a small dose of steroid in women who have had recurrent miscarriage. Routine testing for these factors is not recommended by the Royal College of Obstetricians and Gynaecologists in their latest guideline.

(vii) **Infection** – A one-off bad infection can cause miscarriage, but it is not thought to be the cause of recurrent miscarriage since you would have to consistently have repeated bad infections (flu-like symptoms) every time you had a pregnancy. However, there is some evidence that "Bacterial Vaginosis" has been linked to miscarriage both early and later on in the pregnancy. One study showed that the use of a particular antibiotic (Clindamycin) used after 12 weeks of pregnancy reduced the risk of subsequent miscarriage and preterm birth.

(viii) **Chronic Endometritis** – otherwise known as an inflammatory change of the lining of the womb, often with unknown cause. This may be a reason for implantation failure of the embryo or indeed a cause of recurrent miscarriage. A biopsy of the endometrial lining is required to make the diagnosis, and thereafter treatment with an antibiotic called *Doxycycline* may help to eradicate this. At the present time there is a clinical trial called the CERM trial (Chronic Endometritis and Recurrent Miscarriage Trial) taking place in the UK. Some clinicians may give empirical treatment of Doxycycline (100mg once per day) for 2 weeks before any IVF treatment or indeed after a woman has had recurrent miscarriages, although this is probably best done as part of a clinical trial like CERM.

(ix) **Inherited clotting defects (Thrombophilia screen)** – There is a list of blood tests that can be done looking at whether a woman with recurrent miscarriage has abnormalities with blood that tends to clot excessively. (Without trying to blind you with science – these include Factor V Leiden, Prothrombin Gene Variant, Protein C and S deficiency, Hyperhomocystenaemia and Antithrombin III). Various studies have shown that these abnormalities may be associated with an increased frequency of recurrent miscarriage and in particular late miscarriage. These defects, which are associated with an increased tendency to cause blood clots, **can be treated with a blood thinning injection (such as low molecular weight heparin or *Clexane*)** on a daily basis to prevent blood clots in pregnancy. There is some evidence that such treatment **can reduce** miscarriage rates. Certainly, if you have a history of recurrent miscarriage and / or a family history of blood clots or another family member has tested positive for these factors, ask to be checked.

(x) **Vitamin D Deficiency** – Vitamin D deficiency is

already known to be associated with pre-eclampsia, preterm birth, gestational diabetes, and small babies. It may also be associated with recurrent pregnancy loss and implantation failure. Some authorities have advised assessment of Vitamin D level in women with recurrent miscarriage with a view to supplementation to potentially improve success rates. NICE (National Institute for Clinical Excellence) state that 400 units of Vitamin D daily are required for prevention for Vitamin D deficiency and 800 units daily for treatment of Vitamin D deficiency. Your doctor can do a blood test to see if you are Vitamin D Deficient.

So, what should I do? Our feelings on the matter and generally what happens in real life:

After 1 miscarriage

We wouldn't be inclined to have any tests. Miscarriage is so common that starting a battery of tests after 1 single miscarriage would not be appropriate. We would simply get on with the process of getting pregnant again. The fact that you got pregnant in the first place is reassuring. We would however advise you to take Vit D, Folic Acid (prevents spina bifida), ensure a good diet, stop smoking, avoid alcohol, ensure a healthy weight and get plenty of sleep.

After 2 consecutive miscarriages

Some couples ask to be investigated at this point for fear of the third pregnancy miscarrying, which could have been avoided if investigations and then treatment for any abnormalities had been carried out. We have some sympathy with this chain of thought, particularly if the woman is 35 years old or more when her miscarriage rate is starting to go up anyway and her fertility is starting to reduce. The tests at this point would be the same as for 3 consecutive miscarriages.

After 3 consecutive miscarriages

You need investigation and we would do the following:

(i)   Antiphospholipid screening – blood test.

(ii)   Thyroid Function test and HBA1c (test for diabetes) – both blood tests.

(iii) Vitamin D testing to see if you are deficient.

(iv) Ultrasound scan of the pelvis to ensure normal anatomy.

(v)   Ensure genetic testing of "products of conception" (tissue from your womb following the miscarriage). If this was abnormal then chromosomal analysis of both partners – blood tests for the woman and her partner – is required. This test is only carried out in the NHS at or after 3 consecutive miscarriages.

(vi) Thrombophilia screen – blood test to see if clotting is normal, particularly if one of the miscarriages occurred later than 10 weeks and / or there is a family history of thrombosis (blood clots).

(vii) Biopsy of the endometrium to look for chronic endometritis. (Currently this is being done in a research capacity looking for inflammatory change in the lining of the womb).

In addition, if a late miscarriage (greater than 12 weeks) previously occurred:

(viii) A vaginal swab should be taken when the pregnancy is 10- 12 weeks gestation, to identify "bacterial vaginosis" and if this is present, treat with antibiotics.

(ix) Serial ultrasound scans of the cervical length (length of the neck of the womb) every 1- 2 weeks should be carried out and if this shortens to less than 2.5cm, discussion regarding the insertion of a stitch in the neck of the womb with the couple should be undertaken.

(x) Immune testing is not indicated and the Royal College of Obstetricians and Gynaecologists guidelines agree with this.

So now what treatment is sensible prior to and during an early pregnancy?

1. Regular follow-up and ultrasound scans are reassuring and may help during the course of early pregnancy.

2. Ensure that steps are taken to reduce the patient's BMI to less than 35, ensure that they have stopped smoking if relevant, ensure that they are on Folic Acid (~400 micrograms daily).

3. Advise to ensure no smoking, alcohol or coffee during pregnancy.

4. Supplement their diet with prophylactic Vitamin D (10 micrograms or 400 units daily) – this is present in Pregnacare (specifically designed for pregnancy).

5. If diabetes is picked up, then good control can minimise your risk of miscarriage and future congenital abnormalities.

6. If thyroid disease is identified, treatment with thyroxine is thought to reduce miscarriage rates.

7. If Antiphospholipid screening is positive, then treatment with low-dose aspirin (75mg daily) and a small injection of a low molecular weight heparin (LMWH) such as enoxaparin 40mg daily (otherwise known as Clexane) from conception onwards is thought to be beneficial. Clexane or LMWH are commonly known as "blood thinners" and reduce the incidence of blood clots.

8. If genetic abnormalities are present, then referral to a specialist genetic counsellor is appropriate.

9. There is some evidence that the use of progesterone in early pregnancy either as pessaries (commonly known as Cyclogest or Utrogestan) or injections (Lubion) can help. There have been 2 good quality studies looking at the use of progesterone:

a. PROMISE (Progesterone in Recurrent Miscarriage) study which found higher live birth rate in women using progesterone (400mg *Cyclogest* into the vagina twice per day).

b. PRISM Study (Progesterone in Spontaneous Miscarriage) which also found a higher live birth rate in women using *Cyclogest*.

Certainly, there was no harm associated with the use of progesterone in early pregnancy and since women who present with bleeding in early pregnancy (especially if they have a history of previous miscarriage) may benefit from this, we would recommend the use of Cyclogest 400mg twice per day. It is interesting that NICE (The National Institute for Health and Care Excellence) have recently updated their guidance (Nov 2021) and have essentially agreed that if a woman has bleeding in early pregnancy and has had a previous miscarriage then the use of Cyclogest (400mg into the vagina twice per day) is warranted.

10. If the "thrombophilia screen" (abnormal blood clotting tests) is positive, women can be at risk of thrombosis (clots commonly in the legs and even lungs). Since there is also some evidence that a positive thrombophilia screen is associated with miscarriage, it does not seem unreasonable to use *Clexane* 40mg daily in these women.

11. Some doctors in private clinics use a small dose of steroid (usually prednisolone 5-20mg) in early pregnancy because the theory is that if there is an immunity problem in terms of the pregnant patient's body attacking the pregnancy to cause recurrent miscarriage, then a steroid should reduce that attack, and in doing so theoretically reduce the chance of miscarriage. There is

no overwhelming evidence to support this, and there may be side effects - so careful discussion with your doctor is advised.

12. If there is a congenital abnormality of the womb (for example some women have a partition or "septum" dividing the womb in half), some doctors would recommend surgery to remove the septum or partition. It is thought that approximately 65-85% of patients with this physical abnormality of their womb will have a successful pregnancy after surgery to remove the septum. However, approximately 60% of the same group of women will have a successful pregnancy without surgery and if they continue to try and get pregnant up to around 80% of them will eventually have a live baby. **In addition, a recent study has shown that there is no benefit in surgically removing a septum or partition in the uterus and that such surgery does not improve reproductive outcomes.** Therefore, careful discussion with your doctor is needed, particularly since surgery has its own risks.

13. Intra-uterine adhesions / scar tissue – this can happen following miscarriage treated with – **repeated surgical removal** of retained products (otherwise known as an Evacuation of Retained Products of Conception or ERPOC). It can also occur after an old fashioned "D & C". Scar tissue can form inside the womb and this can be related to pregnancy loss in the future. Such scar tissue or adhesions can be diagnosed with a hysteroscopy (see chapter 4) and scar tissue can be excised at the same time, but there is no guarantee of a successful pregnancy outcome thereafter. Certainly, prevention is better than cure and so in the event of a miscarriage it is better to opt for a medical treatment to manage retained products of conception (in other words, using medication as opposed to surgical removal) or just waiting for your own body to expel the products of conception

(expectant management). However, in the event of excess bleeding and failed medical management, sometimes surgical management is necessary.

So what happens if you have recurrent miscarriage but ALL the tests are normal?

It is not uncommon to have all these tests carried out and they are all normal. If this is the case, the good news is that approximately 75% of the time the next pregnancy will be successful with supportive care alone (in other words regular medical follow-up/ultrasound scans/reassurance). This percentage of course goes down with increasing age, particularly of the mother.

Even if all the tests are negative, many doctors will treat the woman in early pregnancy with the following:

(i) Progesterone pessaries or injections – These help to stabilise the lining of the womb (endometrium) and the theory is that they help to prevent the lining (to which the developing foetus is attached) from coming away. The evidence for this is limited, but certainly there is no evidence that it does any harm.

(ii) Aspirin – For many years some doctors have encouraged the use of low-dose Aspirin (75mg daily) in women who have had miscarriages. There is evidence that it **is useful in women with recurrent miscarriage who have been diagnosed with antiphospholipid syndrome** and in women who have suffered with pre-eclampsia (used to be called toxaemia) in a previous pregnancy. However, in women with **unexplained** recurrent miscarriage syndrome, recent evidence has suggested that Aspirin **is not** helpful and may increase bleeding. Hence, Aspirin does not appear to be of benefit in women with previous unexplained miscarriage, but taken after 12 weeks may reduce the risk of pre-eclampsia, and may be helpful in women with hypertension (high blood pressure), diabetes, a history of a previous abnormally small baby or indeed in women who have suffered the tragedy of a previous still-birth.

(iii) Low Molecular Weight Heparin (LMWH) or Clexane – *Clexane* can very rarely cause thinning of the bones and something called "thrombocytopenia", which in English means it reduces the numbers of tiny little particles in the bloodstream called platelets. These help with the clotting process. This is very rare and the vast majority of women on *Clexane* will have no problems. Some doctors prescribe *Clexane* for women with unexplained recurrent miscarriage syndrome because it is unlikely to cause any harm, and it *may* help. There may be some clotting or immune factor in recurrent miscarriage syndrome that the scientific community is not even aware of, a factor that might be treated with *Clexane*.

(iv) Steroids – To reiterate, some doctors prescribe steroids for women with unexplained recurrent miscarriage syndrome. There may be some immune factor in recurrent miscarriage syndrome that the scientific community is not even aware of, a factor that might be treated with a small dose of steroid, such as Prednisolone 5mg daily. This may be particularly relevant in women who suffer with an inflammatory / immune condition.

(v) Vit D supplementation – 10 micrograms/400 units daily.

(vi) Psychological support with patient support groups, meditation, acupuncture

(vii) Early pregnancy scans

Careful discussion with your doctor regarding the above is essential.

So, the main messages are:

1. Do not wait too long to have your children. The risk of miscarriage goes up with increasing age, especially after 35 years of age.

2. Do not wait too long to have your children. The risk of chromosomal abnormality (for example, Down's syndrome) goes up with increasing age.

3. If you are young and have had 3 miscarriages in a row, you NEED investigation.

4. If you are older, and have had 2 miscarriages in a row, it may not be unreasonable to ask for investigations.

5. Find an empathetic, supportive doctor or clinic. Empirical treatment as above is not unreasonable for patients who feel that they have nothing to lose.

6. Treatment with Progesterone / Clexane / Aspirin / Vitamin D / Early Pregnancy Support / Regular Early Pregnancy Scans / Doxycycline may be indicated – discuss with your doctor.

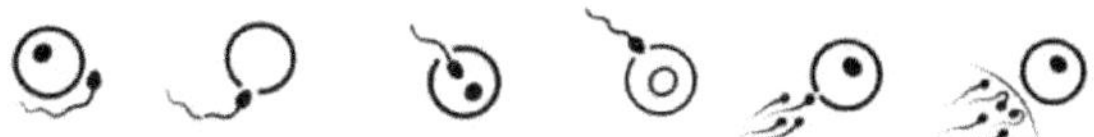

CHAPTER 11

POLYCYSTIC OVARIAN SYNDROME (PCOS)

What is Polycystic Ovarian Syndrome (PCOS)?

This is a condition commonly seen in women who do not have regular periods and who do not ovulate (release an egg) on a regular basis. Hence it is frequently seen in women presenting with infertility. It is the commonest hormonal condition affecting women (approximately 5-10% of the female population). The phrase "polycystic" is an inappropriate name for this condition because the ovaries do not contain "cysts" in the true sense of the word, they merely contain follicles that have stopped growing. A better name would be "Poly-follicular Ovarian Syndrome". The follicles are usually no more than 9mm in diameter, in other words hardly "cystic" (a good going ovarian cyst is 5cm or more) and despite what women are often told, these "Poly-follicular" ovaries do NOT give rise to pain. Ultrasound appearance shows enlarged ovaries with multiple small follicles usually cited peripherally (like a string of beads around the outer part of the ovary).

The definition of PCOS (according to the European Society of Human Reproduction and Embryology) includes 2 out of 3 criteria:

(i)   Infrequent periods (irregular or prolonged times between periods) or anovulation (no ovulation).

(ii) Physical signs of excessive androgens (testosterone) like excessive hair growth/acne or blood tests indicating excessive androgens (testosterone).

(iii) Ultrasound scan evidence of polycystic ovaries.

From the above, you can therefore see that if a woman has polycystic ovaries on ultrasound, but has regular periods and no evidence of excessive hair growth/acne, she does NOT have Polycystic Ovarian *Syndrome* because she only has 1 out of 3 criteria. Women can have polycystic ovaries on ultrasound scan and regularly ovulate.

Are women with polycystic ovaries obese? Does losing weight help to improve their fertility?

It is thought that about 40-50% of PCOS women are obese, so conversely many women with PCOS are relatively slim. This means there is great variability in how PCOS presents. Patients with PCOS may be obese or slim, have problems with excess body hair or not, have problems with acne or have clear skin, may have polycystic ovaries on ultrasound or may not. It is the combination of factors as above that leads to the diagnosis.

It is upsetting for women with PCOS who are obese, that further weight gain can worsen established symptoms of excessive body hair, acne, and irregular periods with reduced chances of ovulation. **Weight loss, on the other hand**, is likely to reduce symptoms of acne, excess body hair, whilst promoting regular periods and even ovulation.

What happens to the hormones in PCOS?

When ordering blood tests, your doctor should include:

(i) Testosterone – levels of this go up in PCOS and this is what causes the increase in body and facial hair together with acne.

(ii) LH – Luteinising Hormone – the level of LH goes up in PCOS in comparison to the level of FSH – Follicle Stimulating Hormone. You will remember from previous chapters that it is the LH surge that is responsible for ovulation. But if the LH is continuously raised there is no surge and there is no ovulation. Therefore be careful interpreting LH ovulation kits that you buy over the counter since a high level of LH may not mean that you have ovulated that month.

(iii) Oestrogen – levels of this hormone are the same or higher in PCOS. Oestrogen causes growth of the lining of the womb (endometrium) in preparation for the embryo to implant.

(iv) Progesterone – you will remember from previous chapters that progesterone is produced by the ovarian follicle that has released an egg and collapses, becoming a "corpus luteum". Progesterone stabilises the lining of the womb that has previously grown under the influence of oestrogen. If it is stopped or withdrawn, then the endometrium no longer is stabilised and breaks down, causing you to have a period. In PCOS, there is no ovulation, hence there is no collapsed follicle or "corpus luteum", hence there is no progesterone production, hence there is no eventual progesterone withdrawal, and so women do not have regular breakdown of the lining of the womb or periods. This means that the lining of the womb can continue to grow under the influence of oestrogen, which can lead to thickened and abnormal changes in the endometrial lining.

(v) AMH – this is usually very high (>35) in patients with PCOS. This means that there are plenty of eggs in the ovaries of patients with PCOS, but they are not being released.

How do you test to see if you are ovulating?

See Chapter 4 (So what investigations do you need?).

How do you treat women with PCOS who are not ovulating?

In describing how to treat patients with PCOS, it is also important to point out that as well as having an increase in androgens (testosterone), PCOS is also characterised by an increase in "Insulin Resistance". This means your liver and fat cells are not as good at using sugar (glucose). That means sugar levels rise which causes your pancreas to produce more insulin. This can lead to pre-diabetes and diabetes. Two of the treatments named below, namely *Metformin* and *Myo-inositol* act to reduce insulin resistance and are therefore beneficial in this regard as well as helping to increase the chances of ovulation. Other medications include:

(i)   *Clomid/Letrozole* – These medications stimulate FSH (Follicle Stimulating Hormone) to increase the chance of ovulation. See chapter 5A

(ii) The use of Gonadotrophin injections like FSH as in IUI/IVF cycles to stimulate the ovaries to grow follicles that produce eggs.

(iii) The use of *Metformin* – This is a tablet form of medication that can stimulate ovulation in women with PCOS and help them achieve regular periods. It may also lower the risk of miscarriage which is increased in patients with PCOS. It is also used to treat type 2 diabetes and so also lowers blood sugar levels in women with PCOS. Metformin is not formally licensed for ovulation induction, but many clinicians use it. Studies suggest that it is less successful at inducing ovulation compared to *Clomid*, but it has the added advantage of helping to reduce weight in obese patients with PCOS as well as improving your chance of ovulating. Side effects include nausea, vomiting, stomach pains, and loss of appetite (approximately 1 in 10 patients) and clinicians are advised to start patients on a low dose and build up. Hence start with 500mg once a day for a week, increase to 500mg twice per day for a week, then 500mg three times a day thereafter. If the higher dose is not tolerated, just use 500mg twice per day. Metformin needs to be taken for approximately 60-90 days before any benefit is noticed.

(iv) *Myo-inositol (Inofolic)* belongs to the Vitamin B complex group has been shown to improve ovulatory function (improves the chances of ovulation in PCOS patients without increasing the risk of twins), reduces insulin resistance, and improves the number and quality (maturity) of eggs collected in IVF cycles. It is both safe and simple to take. It is not a prescription medicine, but can be bought online or from a health food store. There is evidence that it alleviates hirsutism (excess body hair) and reduces acne, as well as having a beneficial effect on a woman's (with PCOS) fertility. We would advocate the use of *Inofolic Alpha* (available at fertilityfamily.co.uk).

(v) Laparoscopic Ovarian Drilling – this is essentially keyhole surgery that then burns little holes in the ovary or ovaries. The way this works is unknown, but it does seem to help with cycle control and stimulate ovulation particularly in patients with high LH levels – ask your doctor.

(vi) If ovulation does not occur with 100mg *Clomid,* there is no evidence that increasing the dose to 150mg is beneficial, *Letrozole* or ovulation induction with gonadotrophins (FSH) would be indicated.

Finally, there is no justification in using Clomid in someone who is already be shown to be ovulating. This may even reduce your chance of becoming pregnant.

Extras you need to know about PCOS

(i)   As already indicated, women with PCOS have something called increased insulin resistance, which means that they are bordering on becoming diabetic. It is also true that women with PCOS are much more likely (10-20% in later life) to become Type 2 diabetics (non-insulin dependent diabetes) in comparison to other women in the general population. Therefore, it is even more important to watch their diet and exercise regularly. Plenty of exercise, a healthy diet, and avoidance of obesity is likely to help act against this trend in middle age. A healthy BMI to aim for is 20-25 – there are BMI calculators on the internet which will tell you your BMI if you input your weight and height. If you do have a raised BMI, even a 5% bodyweight loss can help to make your cycles more regular and improve your chances of pregnancy.

(ii)   Women with PCOS should ensure that they have a period at least once every 3 months. Some women with PCOS do not menstruate for long periods of time, sometimes many months, sometimes even years. The problem with this is that the endometrial lining can continue to grow without ever being shed. Hence abnormal changes can occur, which can lead to an increase in the risk of developing cancer of the endometrial lining. The easiest way to remedy this is to induce a withdrawal bleed by taking a progesterone (such as *Norethisterone* 5mg three times daily) for 10 to 14 days. Once stopped, the endometrial lining is destabilised and the endometrial lining is shed – the woman has a period. Always ensure that you are not pregnant before doing this.

(iii)   When patients with PCOS are stimulated with *Clomid*, there is an increased risk of Ovarian Hyper-stimulation Syndrome (too many follicles stimulated in the ovaries). Stimulation with FSH in women with PCOS undergoing IVF/ICSI/IUI is like an all or nothing phenomenon.

You can stimulate with a low dose of FSH and nothing happens. You increase the dose, then increase it again and still nothing happens – in other words no follicles are produced. You increase it a tiny bit more and "wham" – suddenly tens of follicles appear and the risk of OHSS becomes a reality. So great care is required when stimulating PCOS patients, particularly with FSH.

(iv) If you are not trying to get pregnant sometimes the use of a combined oral contraceptive (COC) pill can be beneficial for the symptoms of PCOS. Particularly if you have resistant acne associated with your PCOS, there is a COC called *Dianette* that can help – ask your doctor.

So, the message is:

1. You may have polycystic ovaries on ultrasound scan, but if you have regular cycles with ovulation with no androgenic features (excess facial or body hair/acne) you do NOT have polycystic ovarian SYNDROME.

2. Obese women with PCOS should be encouraged to lose weight – it will help with cycle control, improve fertility, reduce hirsutism (excess body hair) and help with acne.

3. *Clomid* is a first-line treatment in women with PCOS to help them ovulate. This should be done with regular ultrasound scans (known as Follicle Tracking) to monitor ovarian follicles, give information on timing of ovulation (and therefore sexual intercourse) and ensure no cysts develop.

4. If you are already ovulating there is no point in using *Clomid* which might even be detrimental to your chances of conceiving.

5. If you have PCOS, make sure you have a withdrawal bleed (period) at least once every 3 months unless you are on other hormones that stop your periods (like the contraceptive pill or injection, or the *Mirena* coil).

6. If *Clomid* does not induce ovulation, *Letrozole* may be the next step (although it is unlicensed in the UK). Thereafter, ovulation induction with FSH is the next step.

7. *Inofolic Alpha* is useful in patients with PCOS.

8. *Metformin* should also be considered for regulation of cycles, with improved ovulation and it may help with weight loss induction.

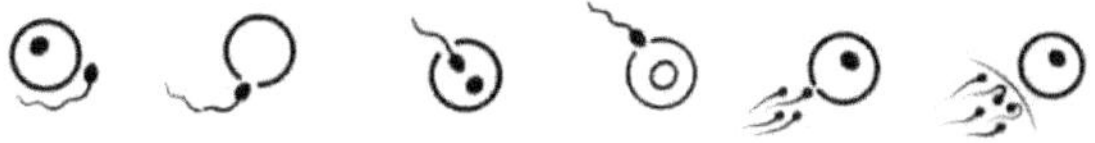

CHAPTER 12

ENDOMETRIOSIS

Endometriosis is associated with reduced fertility and pelvic pain.

What is endometriosis and how common is it in the general population?

First of all, patients often ask, "What is endometriosis?" Despite being diagnosed with it and then told that they have the disease, they do not really understand what it is. In the broadest of layman's terms, endometriosis is essentially the lining of the womb (endometrium) existing and growing outside the womb. This means that in younger women in every cycle that goes by, the endometrium or lining of the womb grows thicker and then sheds as a period or menstrual loss. At the same time any other endometrium (endometriosis) outside the womb and dotted about the pelvis will also grow and shed, causing little bleeds – this can cause "scar" tissue and adhesions (sticky strands) which can then potentially damage the ovaries and fallopian tubes. Also, any scar tends to contract which can cause pulling between ovaries, tubes, and even the bowel – this can result in everything getting stuck together. So the tubes get blocked, the ovaries get covered and sometimes then cannot release eggs properly and patients become infertile AND get pain – pelvic pain which is usually worse during a period and pain during sex.

Endometriosis is very common and thought to affect 10-15% of women of reproductive age, and in those patients presenting to fertility clinics, it is thought to be present in 25-50% of patients.

What causes it?

There are many theories, but the truth is that nobody really knows.

How is it diagnosed?

If a young woman presents with awful pelvic pain, especially if it is cyclical in nature, pain on sexual intercourse, then endometriosis should always be considered. From a gynaecologist's point of view, there are 4 pathological conditions that give a young woman pain in her pelvis:

(i)   Pregnancy – ectopic pregnancy (pregnancy in the tube) or miscarriage

(ii) Pelvic infection – which can cause tubal blockage, pus and abscesses within the pelvis

(iii) Ovarian cysts – but these generally need to be 5cm or more in diameter

(iv) ENDOMETRIOSIS

Other common non-gynaecological reasons for pelvic pain include constipation and cystitis (bladder infection). If the pregnancy test is negative, the swabs show no evidence of infection, and the ultrasound scan of the pelvis shows no cysts… then endometriosis must be considered.

The best way to diagnose endometriosis is to have a laparoscopy (keyhole surgery) – which is basically a fibre-optic camera usually placed through your tummy button (umbilicus) to look inside your pelvis. You need to be put to sleep for this (general anaesthesia). At the same time, the surgeon can surgically treat endometriosis by excising it, burning it off, or using a laser to remove it. Sometimes, endometriosis presents as "chocolate cysts" in one or both ovaries. It is possible to remove these cysts with keyhole surgery, although there is chance that by excising such cysts, healthy (egg-producing) ovarian tissue can also be destroyed in the process.

An ultrasound scan of the pelvis can also help with the diagnosis, but can generally only be used to see "chocolate cysts" of the ovaries. It will not necessarily see the patches of endometriosis that are seen with a laparoscope – so a normal ultrasound scan does NOT exclude endometriosis.

Are there different stages of endometriosis?

Following a diagnostic laparoscopy, endometriosis can be classified as:

(i) Minimal or mild - stages 1-2 – minimal disease with a few superficial implants and some deeper implants.

(ii) Moderate to severe - stages 3-4 – many deep implants, some small cysts on one or both ovaries, and filmy adhesions to large cysts on one or both ovaries and many thick adhesions (or scar tissue) and distorted anatomy.

If endometriosis is present in the ovaries, then bleeding into ovarian cysts occur with the formation of 'endometriomas' or chocolate cysts (so called because the blood contained within the cysts looks like liquid chocolate).

Endometriosis can also grow from the lining of the womb into the muscle of the womb giving heavy painful periods – this is called 'Adenomyosis'.

How does endometriosis cause infertility?

Mild endometriosis is thought to cause an inflammatory response in the pelvis which is thought to impair the function of the ovaries, tubes and endometrium.

Moderate to severe endometriosis often causes distorted anatomy which can block the fallopian tubes, cover the ovaries in adhesions, preventing the proper release of eggs into the tubes, as well destroying ovarian tissue. It will also cause a general "inflammatory" environment within the pelvis which is thought to reduce the chance of pregnancy. Finally, if the pelvis is distorted and sex is painful, the frequency of intercourse may decline, affecting fertility.

Whilst endometriosis can cause reduced fertility, it is also true that many women who have endometriosis successfully conceive naturally. So, a diagnosis of endometriosis does not necessarily equate to an inability to have children. We have on many occasions seen endometriosis at laparoscopy in women having sterilisations because they do not want more children! That having been said, endometriosis does appear to be present in a significant number of women who have problems getting pregnant. However, remember that it is also true that many women with proven fertility also have endometriosis.

Can endometriosis be cured and how is it treated?

Once the diagnosis is made, endometriosis can certainly be effectively treated but it is a chronic and ongoing disease that may well return if the woman is still having menstrual cycles. The growing and shedding of the endometrial tissue whether in the womb or outside the womb (as in endometriosis) is driven by oestrogen produced by the ovaries. Therefore when a woman becomes menopausal and the ovaries stop working, endometriosis gets better. If the ovaries are removed (often with the womb i.e. a hysterectomy), then endometriosis gets better. Oddly, when a woman becomes pregnant, because there is no menstruation (and no variation with no ups and downs of oestrogen levels), endometriosis gets better.

Treatment of endometriosis usually starts with a diagnostic

surgical keyhole procedure (laparoscopy) and removal (excision), ablation (burning off endometriosis). Mild endometriosis can be treated by a general gynaecologist, but if the endometriosis is severe it is better for any surgical treatment to be carried out by laparoscopic surgeon who specialises in the surgical treatment of endometriosis. This is because the surgery can be quite complex. Initial surgical treatment may help with pain and improve fertility.

Following initial diagnosis and surgery, doctors often will give hormonal treatment that stops the cyclical ovarian production of oestrogen, which in turn stops the menstrual cycle (so no growing and shedding of the lining of the womb), which in turn stops the growth of endometriosis. The trouble with giving hormone treatment is that if you stop the menstrual cycle, you will also stop the woman getting pregnant. But commonly used medical treatments for endometriosis include:

I. The combined oral contraceptive pill – this can be taken in the normal way or can be used so that you only have a withdrawal bleed every 3 months by taking 3 packets in a row followed by a 7- day break when a withdrawal bleed occurs.

II. GnRHa (Gonadotrophin Release Hormone analogue) which is either given as a daily nasal spray or an injection (for endometriosis these injections are given every month or even every 3 months in contrast to the daily injections during an IVF cycle). The GnRHa downregulates or stops the production of your own fertility hormones. This therefore makes you temporarily menopausal and by stopping the production of oestrogen will help to treat endometriosis. This treatment is usually very good in sorting out the pain associated with endometriosis and will stop your periods. It is most often given in the form of a monthly injection (*Prostap* or *Zoladex*) for 4-6 months at a time. Side effects can include "hot flushes" as experienced when a woman gets to the menopause and thinning of bones if used for too long. These symptoms can be remedied by using something called 'addback' HRT, a common example is a medication called *Livial.* This protects your bones, alleviates hot flushes and does not seem to cause flare up of endometriosis.

III.   Progesterones – these can be used in the form of the progesterone only pill (POP) such as *Desogestrel* which are used continuously or indeed a promising new treatment called *Dienogest* which is licensed for the treatment of endometriosis (also see later in the chapter with regard to its use prior to an IVF cycle).

Does repeat surgery for endometriosis enhance your chances of having a baby?

Following the initial keyhole surgery to enable a diagnosis and surgical treatment of endometriosis, which may well reduce pain and improve fertility, studies suggest that **repeat surgery (with all its risks) does NOT improve your fertility**. Since endometriosis is a chronic life-long disease, the goal should be to maximise good medical treatment and try and avoid repeat surgery. Repeat surgery may well be accompanied by the formation of yet more adhesions and scar tissue, and many believe it should only be carried out for symptoms of pain.

What is the best fertility treatment in women with endometriosis?

Firstly, remember that many women who have endometriosis still manage to get pregnant and have babies with no problems. After initial surgical diagnosis and treatment if the patient has **minimal/mild endometriosis and all else is normal then options include trying to conceive**

naturally/IUI/IVF – there is no absolute consensus. IVF is the most effective option, but it is much more costly (if the procedure is being done privately), with potentially more side effects. IUI is less effective, and if it is not successful leads to delay in treatment with the more effective option (IVF). To reach the right decision, many factors have to be taken into account that may affect relative success rates. Factors such as a woman's age, whether she has been pregnant before, and whether she has other medical problems. Therefore proper discussion with your IVF fertility specialist is important. For example, in a patient who is 35 years or older, we will often recommend going straight for IVF, because the older you are the more difficult it is to get pregnant and therefore it is important to use the most effective treatment in a timely manner (even if it is more expensive and has more risks associated with it). **For patients with moderate to severe endometriosis, IVF/ICSI is the best option.**

Does endometriosis affect success rates in patients undergoing IVF?

Patients with minimal or mild endometriosis appear to have the same pregnancy and live birth rates when undergoing IVF when compared to patients who do not have endometriosis.

However, although it is controversial, patients with severe disease particularly if they have endometriomas or chocolate cysts on their ovaries **appear to have reduced success rates with IVF.** Endometriosis of the ovaries may well affect the ovarian reserve or the number of eggs. On occasions, particularly if the woman is older with previous failed cycles and severe endometriosis, the use of **IVF with donor eggs is a possible option.**

If you have endometriomas or chocolate cysts on your ovaries – should they be removed before IVF?

If the woman has a chocolate cyst that is less than 4cm most fertility doctors would not request surgery to remove these – removal does not appear to improve outcome and may damage the underlying ovarian tissue. The exception to this is when a chocolate cyst is obstructing the collection of eggs during an IVF egg collection.

Does having IVF worsen your endometriosis?

The answer to this appears to be no, it does not. Going through an IVF cycle does not make your endometriosis worse.

Does treating endometriosis medically help to improve success rates if you are having IVF?

If you are having IVF, pre-treatment with medical therapies (hormone treatment – GNRHa – *Zoladex* or *Prostap*) for 3 months before your IVF treatment to "Downregulate" and treat endometriosis may help improve pregnancy rates, but this is controversial – although some fertility doctors may implement this. There is some evidence that a course of Dienogest (2mg daily) prior to IVF in patients with endometriosis (particularly if they have had previous failed cycles) may help. Dienogest has anti-inflammatory properties and may be worth considering prior to IVF.

Does IUI improve pregnancy rates in mild endometriosis compared to trying naturally?

The simple answer is, "Yes." In women with mild endometriosis and infertility, as long as the fallopian tubes are open there is evidence that stimulated IUI increases the pregnancy rate.

So, the message is:

1. Endometriosis is very common and there should be a low threshold for diagnostic laparoscopy to make the diagnosis.

2. Many women with endometriosis get pregnant and have children and never know that they have it.

3. Surgical treatment of endometriosis appears to help women get pregnant naturally, but does not seem to help improve pregnancy rates if you are having IVF.

4. Hormonal treatment of endometriosis does not seem to help get women pregnant naturally, but hormonal treatment prior to IVF may help increase pregnancy rates.

5. Stimulated IUI cycles in women with endometriosis improves the pregnancy rates.

6. Pregnancy helps endometriosis.

7. If you have pelvic pain/pain on intercourse with no explanation, request a laparoscopy to confirm the diagnosis of endometriosis.

8. If you have moderate or severe endometriosis – make sure that the gynaecologist who does your surgery specialises in endometriosis.

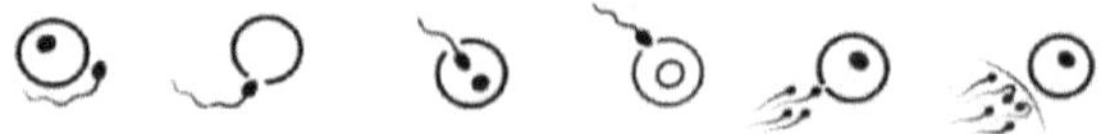

CHAPTER 13

ALL THINGS TO DO WITH SPERM, MALE INFERTILITY AND THE USE OF DONOR SPERM

Approximately a third to half of the time, it is male factor that is the cause of the subfertility or infertility.

What is a Normal Sperm Count?

World Health Organisation (2010) 5th edition

– normal values for Semen Samples:

Volume per ejaculate	1.5ml
Concentration of Sperm	15 million /ml
Progressive Motility	32%
Normal Forms	4%

Historically, the table above (the 5th Edition of the WHO values for a semen sample) sets out what is a normal sample every time a man ejaculates and this is still used by most IVF clinics up and down the UK. However, the WHO have recently produced a 6th edition (2021) with regard to normal values in a sperm test because there is thought to be an overlap in what constitutes normality or abnormality. They still use the same parameters from the table above, namely:

(i) Sperm Concentration – how many millions of sperm per ml

(ii) Motility or Sperm Movement

(iii) Morphology – essentially what the sperm look like – normal or abnormal

Another criterium that is looked at is:

(iv) Sperm Antibody Binding – some men become infertile because they produce antibodies against their own sperm which then clump together and essentially neutralises the sperm's ability to fertilise an egg.

But the recent 6th edition has divided these parameters into whether they are **normal** or **borderline** or frankly **abnormal**. Thus:

WHO 6th edition (2021)	Normal	Borderline	Pathological
Semen Volume	>or=1.4ml		<1.4ml
Sperm Concentration	>or=20 million/ml	10-20 million/ml	<10 million/ml
Progressive Motility	>or= 50%	35-49%	<35%
Normal Forms (Morphology)	>or=14%	4-13%	<4%
Sperm Antibody Binding	<50%	50-79%	>or=80%

So, for some men, what was previously regarded as normal according to the old criteria is now borderline – for example previously if you had a sperm concentration of 15 million/ml, you were deemed to be "normal". The new criteria ascribe a concentration of 15 million/ml into a "borderline" group.

These new categories are an attempt to emphasise that the purpose of the semen examination is not to label a man as either normal or abnormal with regard to their semen analysis, but rather to decide the pathway of further evaluation and treatment. Also, the old WHO 5th edition limits were arbitrary. The creation of a "borderline" group will have significant clinical implications as many men whose sample would previously have been labelled as normal using the 5th edition criteria, will now be classified as "borderline" and therefore be eligible for treatment with IUI/IVF or ICSI, whilst still being offered a hope for natural pregnancy.

Unlike men, at birth a woman has a set number of eggs and these reduce in number as time passes until the menopause, at which point they are completely depleted. On the other hand, men continue to produce a new batch of sperm **every 3 months** for many years and in fact fatherhood has on occasions been achieved by old-age pensioners. Sperm counts can vary depending on whether you have had a recent illness or fever, or even depend on when you last had sex. For example, when asked to produce a semen sample you are advised to abstain for 2-3 days beforehand. This is because you may have a suboptimal sample if you ejaculate too frequently. Likewise, there is a body of opinion that states that if it has been a long time since a previous ejaculation, then although the sperm numbers may be increased, the motility (sperm movement) may be reduced. We will often counsel patients therefore as a general rule to have intercourse every 2-3 days during a woman's most fertile period to achieve the best chance of pregnancy.

It is also important to state that if a recent semen analysis has been tested and is suboptimal, then a repeat semen analysis at a later date is advised before anyone can categorically state that it is abnormal. Why? Because a new batch of sperm is produced every 3 months and if that man had had something as simple as a previous fever or viral illness, it may have affected his sperm. Following any such illness, a new batch of sperm is produced and may be completely normal.

Commonly used terms:

Azoospermia – no sperm seen on semen analysis

Oligospermia – reduced number of sperm seen on semen analysis

Teratospermia – abnormal looking sperm on semen analysis

Asthenospermia – reduced number of motile sperm on semen analysis

After 2 abnormal sperm counts, the patient in question needs (i) examination of his genitals to ensure no abnormality (for example the testicles may be small or even absent) and (ii) the following basic blood tests which will guide the fertility doctor as to why there is little or no sperm in the ejaculate:

1. **FSH / LH** – These hormones are produced by your brain (actually a gland in your brain called the pituitary). They stimulate the testicles to produce sperm and testosterone.

2. **Testosterone** – this is produced by the testicles and is responsible for libido, erectile function, development of muscles and bones mass, etc.

3. **Prolactin** – a hormone also produced by the brain. High levels of prolactin can lead to erectile dysfunction and problems with your sperm count.

   Bearing in mind these blood tests, there are 3 basic reasons for very low numbers of sperm in the Semen-analysis:

(i) **Failure of the brain to produce FSH / LH -** The brain normally sends hormonal signals (FSH and LH) to the testicles stimulating them to produce sperm and testosterone – if there is a problem with the production of these hormones in the brain, then the FSH / LH levels are low and the testicles do not get stimulated. Because the testicles are not stimulated, testosterone production is reduced and there is little or no sperm made. This can be remedied / treated by stimulating the testicles with injections of FSH or its equivalent. Fortunately this condition is relatively rare.

(ii) **Testicular failure.** The testicles will sometimes fail (and on examination will be small or absent), so despite adequate levels of FSH / LH from the brain, the testicles fail to produce both sperm and testosterone. When this occurs, the brain senses there is no testicular activity and tries to compensate by pushing out yet more FSH / LH in an attempt to further stimulate the failing testicles. Hence if the FSH / LH is abnormally **high** and testosterone abnormally **low,** it is an indication of testicular failure.

(iii) **Absent or blocked male tubes (which take sperm from the testicles to the penis).** If the tubes are blocked or absent, FSH / LH / Testosterone levels still remain normal, the testicles still produce normal quantities of sperm, but because there is a blockage of the tubes (for example, because the individual has had a vasectomy or indeed because of genetic factors or infection) there is no sperm in the ejaculate.

In addition to the basic blood tests FSH, LH, Prolactin and testosterone, the individual with poor sperm counts (less than 5 million per ml), should also have the following **genetic testing:**

Karyotype – this is a blood test that looks at the chromosomes or genetic material of the individual concerned, especially the 2 chromosomes that determine the biological sex of the individual which are the X and the Y chromosomes. Biological women have two X chromosomes – hence are XX, whereas men have one X chromosome and one Y chromosome – hence XY. Men with a severe reduction in sperm count or no sperm at all in the ejaculate (azoospermia), have an increase in the risk of genetic abnormality. For example, "Klinefelter Syndrome" is a condition in which the individual has an extra X chromosome (hence XXY) and the sperm count is markedly abnormal.

Y-Chromosome Microdeletion – this is another genetic test associated with very low sperm counts which highlights an abnormality of the Y chromosome and is called a microdeletion (part of the chromosome is missing). Approximately 1-30% of cases of men with testicular failure have Y-Chromosome microdeletion.

Cystic Fibrosis Screening – Please see later paragraph on Obstruction / absence of the male tubes.

What lifestyle factors can impair the production of sperm?

Avoid recreational drugs (for example – marijuana, heroin) since they can adversely affect sperm production. **Anabolic steroids may build big muscles but they trash the testicles.** (This occurs by switching off the pituitary gland in your brain, which stops sperm production and in turn leads to shrinking of your testicles.)

Excess alcohol can lower testosterone levels and impair the production of sperm. It can also reduce sex drive and lead to impotence. So, cessation of heavy drinking can make a difference, although it is important to allow time for improvement (at least 3 months).

Likewise, cigarette smoking reduces fertility for him and her, so it's important to stop. Obesity and related diabetes, or any chronic illness for that matter, can impair sperm production –

so lose weight and seek comprehensive treatment for any ongoing illness.

Cycling – there have been reported cases of men spending too much time on the saddle who end up with impaired sperm samples and this reverses when they stop cycling. If the testicles are exposed to too much heat for example, tight-fitting trousers/tight underpants or too many hot baths, there may be impairment of sperm production.

What medical reasons are there for an impaired sperm count?

Undescended Testes

Some men suffer from undescended testicles or "cryptorchidism" to give it its proper medical title. About 3% of male infants have no palpable testicles in the scrotal sac at birth, although most of those have descended by the age of 1 year old.

Some male children have "retractile" testes that can be milked down into the scrotum where they remain for a few seconds before springing back up. Whereas a truly undescended testicle can sometimes be milked down, but will immediately spring back. In cases where the undescended testes do not respond to hormones, surgery (known as "orchidopexy") is required. Men who have had 1 undescended testis tend to be fertile, albeit with a reduced sperm count. Men with a history of both testes undescended are at risk of infertility. It is also important to note men with a history of undescended testes are at greater risk of testicular cancer particularly if they do not have surgery before the age of 10.

Viral Illness

Mumps can cause an "orchitis" (infection/inflammation of the testicles) that can result in infertility. Hence the MMR vaccine protects against this. Other viral illnesses, particularly if they produce a fever, may temporarily affect sperm production.

STDs (sexually transmitted disease)

Not only can chlamydia cause blockage of the fallopian tubes in women, but infection can also cause blockage/damage to the male tubes (epididymis and vas) carrying sperm from the testicle to the penis as well as damage to the testicle itself. Other STDs such as gonorrhoea, which is thankfully less common now than it used to be, can also cause blockage and infertility. Hence the advice for young men and women – *any doubt, use a condom if in a new relationship or having casual sex.*

Varicose Veins of the Scrotum (Varicocele)

Varicose veins in the scrotal sac or varicoceles occur in up to 20% of the male population and feel like a bunch of worms in the scrotum – so they are common. What is interesting is that varicoceles are present in 30-40% of men attending fertility clinics and there is some evidence that they are associated with subfertility. That having been said, many men with varicoceles are fertile. The whole issue about treatment is controversial and there is no overwhelming evidence that surgery/treatment improves male fertility.

Trauma/Chemotherapy/Radiotherapy

Trauma is an obvious cause for permanent damage to the testicles and care should be taken when playing contact sports in particular.

If a patient has cancer and needs chemotherapy or radiotherapy, it is likely to affect their fertility and ***they should at least be made aware of the possibility of giving sperm samples that can be frozen and then stored for future use before any such treatment.***

Obstruction or Absence of the Male Tubes

About 50% of men with azoospermia (no sperm in the semen sample) actually have normal sperm production in the testicles but there is a blockage preventing the sperm from exiting. This can be due to blockage of the sperm tubes (epididymis/vas) due to infection or previous vasectomy, or failure of the sperm tubes to ever develop (known as congenital absence of the vas deferens – CAVD). About 66% of men with absence of the vas deferens carry the **Cystic Fibrosis** (CF) gene and therefore may require genetic testing for this. If they are positive and carry the gene, then their partner also should be tested to ensure that they too are not carriers. If both the man and woman are carriers of the CF gene, then potentially any resulting child has a 1 in 4 chance of actually having the disease and 1 in 2 will themselves be carriers. Such couples can still undergo IVF/ICSI, but any resultant embryos can be tested with PGD (Pre-implantation Genetic Diagnosis) whereby 1 or 2 cells from each embryo are tested for the CF gene and only the embryos that are normal are then replaced. This ensures the CF gene isn't passed on to any resultant children.

Testicular Failure with no obstruction of the Male Tubes

Approximately 50% or more men with very poor sperm samples will not necessarily have an obstruction of the male tubes, but have testicles that just do not work or produce very few sperm. Such patients will require genetic testing in the form of a Karyotype, Y Chromosome Micro-deletion tests as described at the beginning of the chapter.

Infertility caused by testicular failure can be overcome with treatment in the form of ICSI even if there are just a few sperm in the ejaculate. Alternatively, if there are no sperm in the ejaculate, they can have a Surgical Sperm Retrieval (SSR), which essentially attempts to surgically remove any sperm from the testicle or male tubes. Again, even with just a few sperm, treatment with ICSI can be successful.

It is important to be aware and ask about any genetic defect which may be transferred from father to son and sometimes referral to a genetic counsellor is wise.

Anti-sperm Antibodies (ASAs)

On occasions when a semen analysis is carried out and the sample is looked at under the microscope, clumping together of the sperm is seen under the microscope, indicating the presence of antibodies. These antibodies can be tested for. Antibodies to the sperm are likely to affect motility and perhaps fertilisation. At least 50% of men who have had a vasectomy will develop antibodies against their own sperm, but also infection, trauma, and the CAVD (Congenital Absence of the Vas Deferens) can cause antibodies against the sperm to form. It is NOT possible to wash off these antibodies and the best option for men with antibodies is to have IVF with ICSI. The concentration of anti-sperm antibodies does not affect success rates and birth rates using ICSI in men with ASAs are the same when compared to couples having ICSI when there are no male infertility problems. Clinicians used to use steroids to treat this – although these days most couples will opt for ICSI.

DNA Fragmentation

As well as the semen analysis test, some clinics may also carry out a "DNA Fragmentation" test – an additional test that looks specifically at any damage to the genetic material in the sperm. It has been estimated that up to 15% of patients with normal semen analysis may still have male infertility, and you would not necessarily know about abnormal sperm DNA from the basic semen analysis test. In addition, if there is significant damage to sperm DNA then natural conception and IUI is very unlikely to be successful. Success rates too with IVF may be reduced and the likely best treatment is ICSI. Fortunately, there is some good news insofar as there is some evidence that the use of anti-oxidants such as vitamin C, vitamin E, selenium, coenzyme Q10, N-acetylcysteine, zinc, and L-carnitine may be effective in reducing DNA fragmentation, which in turn may improve pregnancy rates. However, much more study still needs to be done – but certainly the use of these anti-oxidants is unlikely to do any harm and may help.

Idiopathic Male Factor Infertility (nobody knows)

About 50% of time no reason can be found for abnormal sperm and it is therefore labelled "idiopathic" – this is essentially akin to "Unexplained Infertility". Nobody knows why. Fortunately, it can treated with IVF/ICSI.

If I have Male Factor Infertility... what can be done about it?

Simple Everyday Lifestyle Changes

Basic and obvious lifestyle changes like ensuring no excess alcohol, avoidance of recreational drugs, stopping smoking, eating a good diet of fresh fruit and vegetables, maintaining a healthy weight. All these will not only help with your general health but may also help you to ensure healthy sperm. Ensure protection against STDs – use a condom. Get vaccinated with MMR early in your life. Generally avoiding very hot baths or hot-tubs for prolonged periods is sensible, since the scrotal sac is designed so that testicular temperature is lower than normal body temperature.

Anti-oxidants

We are often asked if there is any evidence with regard to the taking of supplements like zinc, selenium, vitamins B, C, E, and co-enzyme Q10. As indicated above they may be useful if taken in the recommended way and there is no evidence that these supplements will do any harm.

Varicose Veins (Varicocele) of the Scrotum

The evidence is not entirely clear and there are plenty of men with varicoceles who have fathered children. In the UK most surgical treatment is aimed at those who have symptoms, rather than to improve the sperm count especially when IVF/ICSI is available if the sperm count is low.

Chemotherapy/Radiotherapy

If at all possible, have sperm samples collected and frozen to be stored for future use *prior* to any treatment. This means the ability to have children in the future is preserved.

Vasectomy

Vasectomy ("the snip") is essentially division of the vas or sperm tube. Sperm continues to be made by the testicle but cannot be transported beyond the surgically induced blockage.

If a man who has had a vasectomy meets a new partner and they wish to have their own children, there are 2 courses of action available:

1. Surgical Reversal of vasectomy (re-joining of the vas). Approximately 85% of the time a vasectomy can be reversed; the earlier after vasectomy that this reversal is done the better. The longer the time gap between the vasectomy and its reversal the worse the pregnancy rate. Approximately 50% of couples will conceive after reversal of vasectomy.

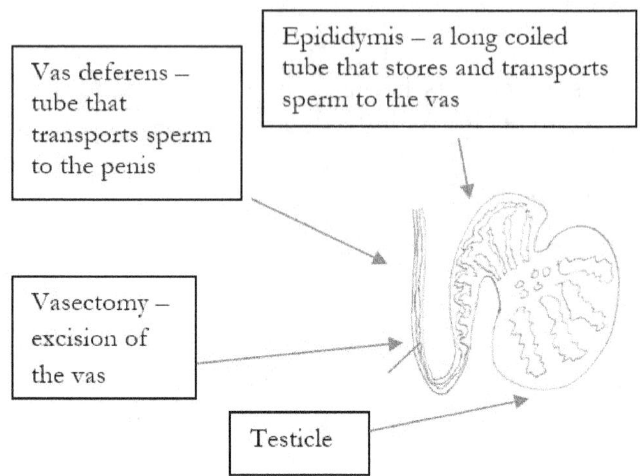

Overcoming Obstruction of the Male Tubes (including vasectomy) / Testicular Failure

A problem with vasectomy is that 50-80% of men develop antibodies against their own sperm – Anti-Sperm Antibodies (ASAs) – these antibodies can cause clumping and affect the motility of the sperm as well as make it difficult for the sperm to interact with the egg – affecting fertilisation. Treatment options include the use of steroids which dampen down the immune system and so reduce the antibody number, OR consider IUI/IVF/ICSI.

2. Surgical Sperm Retrieval (SSR):

PESA (Percutaneous Epidydimal Sperm Aspiration)

TESE/TESA (Testicular Sperm Extraction/Aspiration)

MESA (MicroEpididydimal Sperm Aspiration)

All 3 of these techniques involve either using a needle or a small incision to obtain sperm either proximal to the vasectomy or other blockage. Alternatively, a SSR is used to obtain even very small numbers of sperm directly from a poorly functioning testicle (even when there is no blockage). Any resultant sperm obtained can then be used for ICSI where only 1 good sperm is required and injected per egg collected from the female partner. A fallback position is obviously to use donor sperm.

Surgical Sperm Retrieval

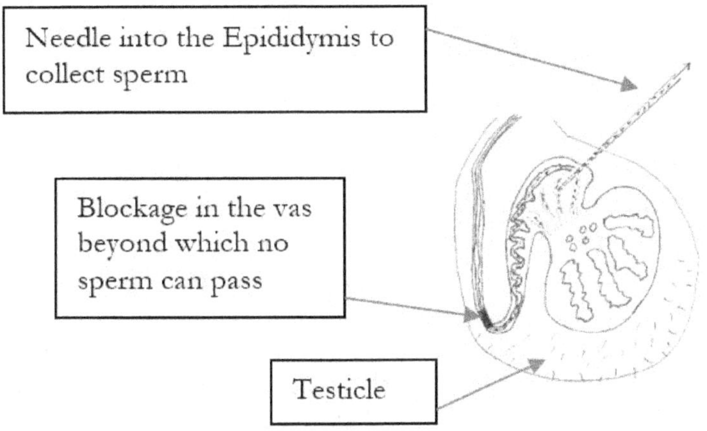

Prior to the SSR, the patient needs to have shaved the scrotum. The procedure is usually done under local anaesthesia often with intravenous sedation and intravenous analgesia (painkillers). There is a risk of infection, bleeding, and bruising and it is sensible to wear supportive underwear following the procedure (no boxer shorts). Aspirin can increase the amount of bleeding and it is therefore sensible not to take aspirin either before or after the SSR.

SSR can be used to obtain sperm following a vasectomy, but also in cases where there is blockage for other reasons, or if there is an absent vas (as in CAVD – congenital absence of the vas deferens), as in patients who carry the CF gene. In addition, it can be tried in patients with azoospermia and testicular failure. In order to predict the likely success of a SSR, a blood test for male FSH or Follicle Stimulating Hormone is carried out. In males, FSH stimulates the production of sperm in the testicles. If this is within the normal range, it is more likely that SSR will be successful.. On the other hand, if it is abnormal then it is less likely that the testicles will be producing sperm and so SSR is less likely to be successful and donor sperm may be a more sensible option.

What happens if I cannot get an erection/ejaculate?

About 20% of the time, this is because of psychological problems like anxiety and depression. The rest of the time there is a physical cause. These include diabetes, multiple sclerosis, spinal cord injury, or previous surgery to the groin area (for example prostate surgery). Some drugs, for example blood pressure tablets or antidepressants can also be responsible. It is sensible to see your GP regarding this as a first line. Your GP can carry out simple screening tests for example, for diabetes, as well as a review of your medication that could potentially exacerbate this problem. Treatment is usually with a group of drugs known as Phosphodiesterase type 5 (PDE5) inhibitors of which '*Viagra*' is an example. If this does not work referral to hospital is appropriate.

What is Retrograde Ejaculation?

Retrograde ejaculation occurs during sex, when instead of the sperm coming out of the end of the penis, it goes into the bladder (the reservoir for urine). This results in only a small amount of sperm being produced externally. The best way to determine the diagnosis is to collect a urine sample after ejaculation. If sperm are seen in the urine, the diagnosis is made. This does make it difficult to achieve a pregnancy naturally, however, if required the sperm can be collected from the urine and used for IVF/ICSI to achieve pregnancy.

This can be found in some people who suffer from diabetes.

If all else fails, what else can I do? DONOR SPERM

Donor sperm is available from various clinics up and down the UK. Sperm can also be imported from overseas, for example:

(i) European Sperm Bank which is based in Denmark (www.esb.com)

(ii) Xytex which is based in the USA (www.xytex.com)

Sperm from these overseas sources have a vast selection of donor sperm available to meet the personal criteria required in terms of characteristics of the donors. They also comply with UK laws regarding screening and quarantining.

Donor sperm can be used not only in the absence of sperm of a partner, but also in cases when the male partner has an inherited condition that the couple do not want to pass on to their children. Remember however, that if there is an inherited condition like Cystic Fibrosis, then a man may use his own sperm together with PGD (Pre-Implantation Genetic Diagnosis) to ensure the resultant embryo that is replaced is free of that condition.

Donor sperm can also be used by same-sex couples, or indeed a single woman who wishes to have a baby but has no male partner.

Donated sperm can used in either IUI or IVF cycles.

When donated sperm is used, your clinic must sort out various consents to enable legality of parenthood for:

(i) Married couples

(ii) Civil partners

(iii) Women who are not married or in a civil partnership but have a male partner

(iv) Women who are not married or in a civil partnership but have a female partner

Certainly, by law the sperm donor will NOT be treated as the father of any child resulting from the use of his sperm in the treatment of others.

In the UK, can children who have been conceived through the use of donor sperm access information about the donor?

The answer to this is yes, once the child is 18 years old (if the donation was made after April 2005). This information can be identifying information including name, date of birth, address, and physical appearance.

In addition, once 18 years old, an individual can also find out about donor-conceived genetic brothers or sisters – if both sides consent.

In the UK, can donors access information about their genetic offspring?

The answer is yes, but the information is anonymous – so they are made aware of the number, sex, date of birth, of people born as a result of their donation.

The Human Fertilisation & Embryology Authority (HFEA) keep a confidential register of all sperm, egg, and embryo donations. This includes information on ethnicity, physical appearance, occupation and interests. The register also includes information on all treatments and children born as a result of such treatments.

Should fertility units offer counselling regarding the use of donor sperm/eggs?

The answer is of course yes. Clinics should offer couples

counselling regarding all aspects of fertility, but particularly the use of donor sperm and eggs.

Further reading, particularly regarding the legal aspects of using donor sperm, can be found on the HFEA website at http://www.hfea.gov.uk.

So, the message is:

1. Poor or absent sperm is responsible for a third to a half of all cases of infertility.

2. The most important investigation for the male partner is the semen analysis or sperm count test.

3. Simple lifestyle changes like avoidance of excess alcohol, stopping smoking, stopping drugs, prevention of STDs, and promotion of loose-fitting clothes can make a difference and are worth trying.

4. The use of dietary supplements like vitamin C, vitamin E, zinc, selenium, Co-enzyme Q10, may be helpful.

5. If positive, a DNA fragmentation test of the sperm may indicate that ICSI is the best treatment going forward.

6. If you have had a vasectomy or there is a blockage or absence of the sperm tubes, sperm can still be retrieved using a surgical sperm retrieval for use with ICSI. If there is no sperm (azoospermia) because of testicular failure, it may still be worth trying surgical sperm retrieval to obtain a few sperm for use with ICSI.

7. If you carry a faulty gene (like Cystic Fibrosis), it is still possible to have your own healthy child, after genetic testing of your partner and any resultant embryos you both produce.

8. If all else fails, you can still use donor sperm.

9. If you are in a same-sex female relationship, you can use donor sperm.

10. If you are a single woman, you can use donor sperm.

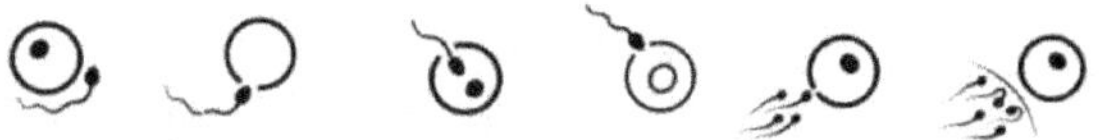

CHAPTER 14

BASIC EMBRYOLOGY –
WHAT YOU NEED TO KNOW

A book on infertility and IVF would not be complete without some mention of the science behind Assisted Reproduction and how it relates to you in your attempts to have a child.

What is an embryologist and what do they do?

An embryologist is a highly trained and specialised scientist who works in the laboratory of IVF Units. They are essentially involved in everything from the basic sperm tests (semen analysis) to identification of eggs at egg collection, to the IVF/ICSI procedure itself when they are responsible for the fertilisation of the eggs, the culturing of the embryos, and the embryo transfer. They are responsible for the storage of sperm/eggs/embryos. Not only do they provide scientific expertise based in the laboratory but they also liaise and provide information to infertile couples both before, during, and after a fertility treatment.

What happens during the development of an embryo during an IVF/ICSI cycle and when is the best time to put an embryo back into the womb?

Day 0 – Egg collection is carried out and the eggs prepared for IVF or ICSI. Sperm is prepared either from a thawed frozen sample or a fresh sample. In IVF up to 150,000 sperm are placed with each egg retrieved. In ICSI 1 sperm is injected into each egg retrieved.

Day 1 – The embryologist carries out a fertilisation check to assess whether the formation of embryos has taken place. The couple concerned are contacted to inform them of the number of fertilised eggs (embryos) achieved.

Day 2 – The embryos have started to divide and are now composed of between 2-4 cells. At this stage the embryo can either be transferred into the womb (Embryo Transfer – ET) or frozen for a Frozen Embryo Transfer (FET) at a later date or be allowed to continue to develop. Day 2/3 embryo transfers are typically for patients with lower embryo numbers (often less than 3 – when there is no perceived benefit to help selection in growing them for longer). Day 2 and day 3 embryos can be graded based on:

(i) How many cells they have,

(ii) How symmetrical these cells are, and

(iii) Whether any fragments (debris) are between the cells.

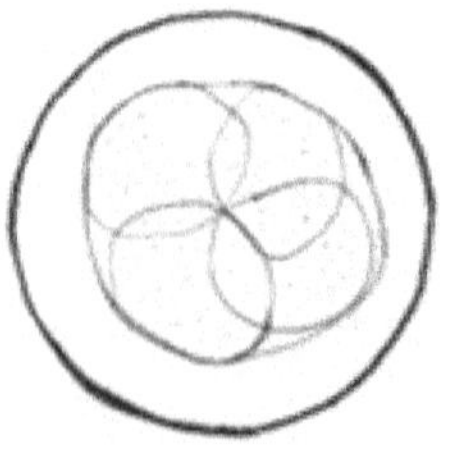

Day 3 – The embryo continues to divide and is now composed of 6-8 cells. At this stage the embryo can either be transferred into the womb (ET) or frozen for a future FET or be allowed to continue to develop to day 5 (Blastocyst stage).

Day 4 – At this stage the embryo is called a Morula. It is just a cluster of cells and as such it is blurry and difficult to grade.

Day 5/6 – The embryo reaches the "Blastocyst" stage. Now the embryo has an "inner cell mass" which will develop into the baby, and the "trophectoderm" which develops into the placenta or afterbirth. The embryo expands to have a fluid-filled cavity and the embryo is encased within a shell through which it must hatch in order to implant into the lining of the womb. Day 5 embryos can be graded based on how expanded (inflated) they are and the appearance of the inner cell mass and trophectoderm.

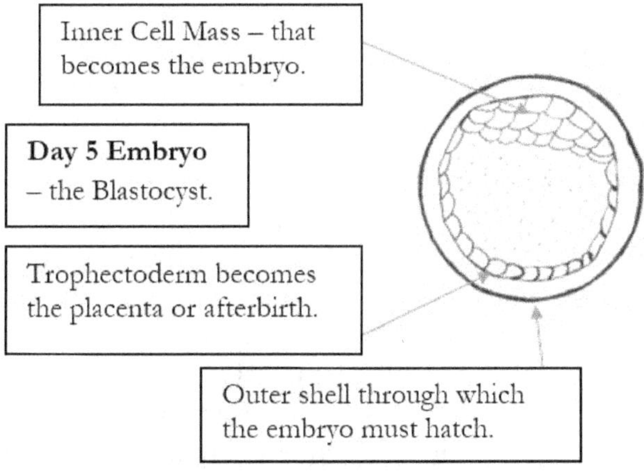

The embryologist grades each embryo to determine the best one or two to place into the womb. As can be seen from the above diagram, there is an outer shell around the embryo from which the embryo needs to hatch in order to implant into the lining of the womb. If the outer shell looks tough, or there is a history of previously failed implantation (especially in the over 40s), then the embryologist can facilitate "hatching" by making a small hole in the outer shell with a laser:

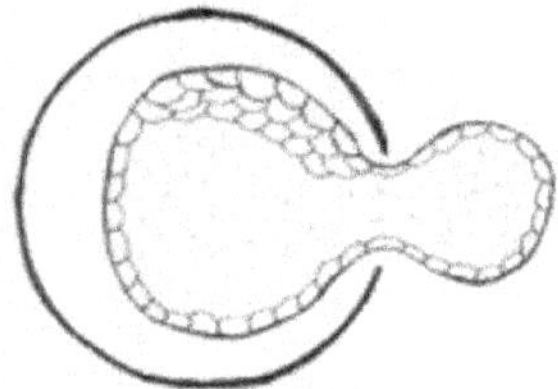

> **Day 5 Embryo –** hatching through its outer shell.

Are there any risks with Assisted Hatching?

If the embryologist undertakes assisted hatching by making a small hole in the outer shell with a laser, there is very little risk to the embryo, if any. There is however, a slight increase in the risk of identical twins (about 1%).

Why wait until day 5 (blastocyst) to put the embryo(s) back?

As already stated, the embryos can be replaced into the womb on day 2/3 or day 5. There is no doubt that the best place for the embryos is in the mother's womb, however the optimum time to judge which are the best embryos likely to result in an ongoing pregnancy is at the blastocyst stage (day 5). Many embryos will die before they reach day 5, but because you do not know which embryos will survive you may carry out embryo transfer using the embryos that would never have survived until day 5. Since only the strongest and best embryos make it to blastocyst and it is these that are replaced into the womb, it is not surprising that pregnancy rates have gone up with blastocyst replacement.

Following on from this, if your egg collection and subsequent fertilisation only results in 2 embryos, it is sensible to have embryo transfer on day 2/3 since there is no choice between embryos and no advantage in waiting until day 5 to replace them. However, if you have more embryos to choose from, wait until day 5 to determine the fittest and the highest grade embryo(s) to replace.

What is a Timelapse Incubator (Embryoscope) and how does it help in choosing the best embryos?

The "embryoscope", which is an example of a timelapse incubator, is a cutting-edge embryo incubator that essentially employs timelapse photography to film the progress of the developing embryos. Traditionally, to see how embryos were developing, an embryologist would remove them from the safety of an incubator to look at them under the microscope – this potentially exposes the embryos to stress and damage. In addition, it can only be done a limited number of times. In contrast the embryoscope takes time-interval photographs (approximately 12 photos per embryo every 12 mins or so) within the safety of the incubator, and the development of each embryo from the time of fertilisation to the time of embryo transfer is recorded.

Hence, when each embryo is ready to be placed back into the womb not only can the embryo be graded according to what it looks like now, but also the development of each embryo from the earliest stages can be assessed. If there has been abnormal development noted by reviewing images from the embryoscope, then that embryo is less likely to produce a viable pregnancy. On the other hand, if the embryo has shown normal development as witnessed by the embryoscope, then it is more likely to yield a viable pregnancy. In this way the embryoscope provides more information on how to choose the best embryos for embryo transfer to improve the chance of a positive pregnancy test and ongoing pregnancy. More recent developments include the use of artificial intelligence (AI) in the lab embryoscope in which computer software identifies patterns of development that the human eye cannot detect based on data from thousands of timelapse embryos that have subsequently implanted. Identification of such patterns of embryo development will hopefully improve success rates with regard to choosing the correct embryos for transfer.

What is Embryo Glue?

The embryos can be placed into "Embryo Glue" prior to their transfer into the womb. This is a great marketing name, but is certainly nothing like glue. It is thought the Hyaluronic Acid ("glue") facilitates communication between cells and is helpful for the process of implantation. There is evidence that this improves pregnancy rates and hence its utilisation prior to embryo transfer.

Embryologists and Sperm Assessment and Preparation

Embryologists carry out semen analysis to determine whether the sperm sample is adequate for IUI or IVF or ICSI, and of course they prepare the sperm for each of these treatments. Sperm preparation involves washing the sperm to remove any dead sperm or debris, then centrifuging or spinning the sperm cells down to increase the concentration. In patients having ICSI, they choose the best sperm and then inject the sperm directly into the collected egg. Historically the embryologist may have offered couples having ICSI, a screening procedure for choosing the best sperm – a procedure called IMSI – please see below:

What is IMSI?

IMSI stands for Intracytoplasmic Morphologically selected Sperm Injection. In English, this means that when the embryologist is looking for the best single sperm to use for injection, they use a special microscope that is x6000 more powerful to assess each sperm. In this way tiny defects in the sperm that would not ordinarily have been seen are detected and only "perfect" sperm used to inject into the egg. The procedure is intended to improve pregnancy success rates and reduce miscarriage rates. However, there is lack of robust evidence to suggest the benefit of IMSI although there are some observational studies which showed improved pregnancy rates and reduction in miscarriage rates. Recent Cochrane review (which roughly translated means 'a respected scientific evaluation of the situation') does not support or refute the clinical use of IMSI. The HFEA has red lighted IMSI as an "add on" because there are doubts about its effectiveness. However, there may be some patients in whom it could be considered and thorough discussion with your fertility consultant is required.

.

What is "DNA Fragmentation" of the sperm?

The head of the sperm contains genetic material called DNA which needs to remain intact. If this genetic material or DNA gets damaged or "fragmented", it may cause problems with subsequent embryos that are produced, both in terms of implantation and possible miscarriage. A "DNA fragmentation test" is essentially a method of looking at the sperm head to determine if there is any genetic damage or fragmentation. Significant DNA fragmentation has been found to reduce pregnancy rates and if this is present IUI is unlikely to work, and ICSI is likely to be better than IVF. This is because in ICSI the embryologist can choose the most normal and best moving sperm to be injected, whilst in IVF the sperm that enters the egg is randomly selected. If there is significant DNA fragmentation in the sperm IUI is unlikely to work. Certainly, if there have been problems in trying to conceive or a lack of success with IVF, a DNA fragmentation test may help and ICSI may be indicated.

Family History of Genetic Abnormality – what can be done to stop the abnormality being passed on?

The answer is PGD or Pre- Implantation Genetic Diagnosis – (now known as PGT-M / PGT-SR)

This is similar to PGS (Pre-implantation Genetic **Screening**) as discussed in Chapter 9, but instead of a general screening for potential parents with no family history of a genetic disorder, in PGD the embryos are tested for a specific **known genetic disorder.**

In English, this means that if there is a genetic abnormality that runs through the family, during the process of IVF or ICSI, after the egg collection and formation of any embryo(s), a cell or cells are taken from the embryo(s) and examined for that specific genetic condition. Thereafter, only the good embryo(s) that are free from the condition are placed back into the womb. There are about 600 conditions that can be tested for – so if a genetic disease runs in the family, it can potentially be avoided in future generations. Some clinics will have this facility. Certainly if a genetic abnormality runs through your family ask your fertility doctor about PGD.

There is more information on this from the HFEA website (www.hfea.gov.uk)

So, the message is:

1. The embryologist is a highly trained scientist working in IVF units who is responsible for all the laboratory aspects of IVF and ICSI.

2. If you have enough embryos, embryo transfer at the Blastocyst stage, day 5, yields higher pregnancy rates.

3. Consider assisted hatching if your embryologist recommends it, particularly if you are over 40 years old or had previous implantation failures.

4. The embryoscope timelapse is useful for better selection of embryos to be transferred.

5. DNA fragmentation tests indicate damage to sperm and it is likely that in such cases ICSI is a better treatment than IVF.

6. IMSI has gone out of favour even if there has been previous implantation failure in an ICSI cycle or when the sperm analysis has shown many sperm with abnormal shape or form. Discuss with your Embryologist before consideration.

7. If you have a family history of a genetic abnormality, Pre-implantation Genetic Diagnosis can be used to ensure only good embryos are placed back in the womb.

ABOUT THE AUTHORS

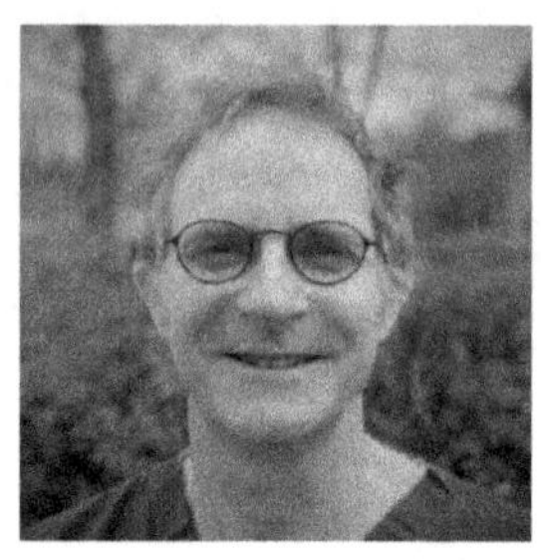

Dr Sean Watermeyer has been an NHS Consultant Gynaecologist for over 15 years, and prior to that was a GP in the Royal Air Force. He has worked in fertility for 20+ years. In his spare time, he writes humorous medical fiction about the antics and adventures of a young gynaecologist (includes *"Medics, Minis & Mayhem"* and its sequel, *"Hospital Blues"*), as well as children's rhyming picture books. He lives in the capital city of Wales with his wife and a golden Labrador called 'Beano'.

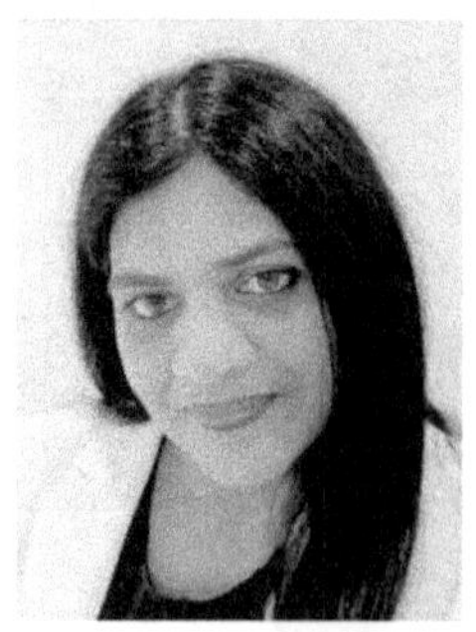

Dr Vidyalatha Atluri has been a fertility consultant for nearly 10 years. She had postgraduate training in obstetrics and gynaecology with special interest in infertility. She worked in different training hospitals all over Northern Ireland. She has been a member of the RCOG since 2005. She is currently working as a fertility consultant at CRGH, London. She lives with her husband and son who remain ever grateful for the other love of her life, cooking.

www.ingramcontent.com/pod-product-compliance
Lightning Source LLC
Chambersburg PA
CBHW051108050726
47592CB00002B/724